BEAT ARTHRITIS NATURALLY

To the other two people who make our three musketeers:

my mum and sister.

BEAT ARTHRITIS NATURALLY

Supercharge your health with
65 recipes and lifestyle tips from
Arthritis Foodie

Emily Johnson

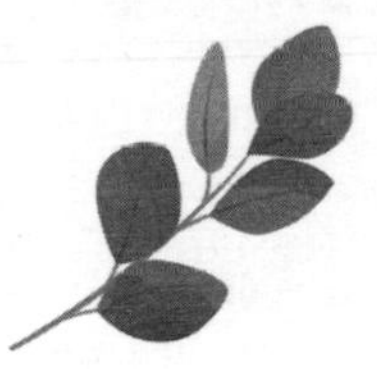

The information in this book is not intended to replace or conflict with the advice given to you by your GP or other health professional. All matters regarding your health should be discussed with your GP or other health professional. The author and publisher disclaim any liability directly or indirectly from the use of the material in this book by any person.

First published in Great Britain in 2021 by Yellow Kite
An Imprint of Hodder & Stoughton
An Hachette UK company

3

Logo by Kate Larsen Design & Illustration

A CIP catalogue record for this title is available from the British Library

Trade Paperback ISBN 978 1 529 34769 2
eBook ISBN 978 1 529 34770 8

Typeset in SABON MT by Manipal Technologies Limited

Printed and bound in Great Britain by Clays Ltd, Elcograf S.p.A.

Hodder & Stoughton policy is to use papers that are natural, renewable and recyclable products and made from wood grown in sustainable forests. The logging and manufacturing processes are expected to conform to the environmental regulations of the country of origin.

Yellow Kite
Hodder & Stoughton Ltd
Carmelite House
50 Victoria Embankment
London EC4Y 0DZ

www.yellowkitebooks.co.uk

Contents

Foreword

Emily Johnson is the founder of Arthritis Foodie, the international health and lifestyle blog dedicated to living well with arthritis. Bringing together numerous health practitioners, including me, *Beat Arthritis Naturally* provides you with vital information you need to know about your arthritis, helping you to make the lifestyle changes required to manage life with your condition, and improve and possibly beat the pain and symptoms.

As a rheumatologist, I see all types of patients with rheumatic diseases at varying stages, including autoimmune diseases and chronic inflammatory conditions. The manifestation of arthritis is a spectrum, and every individual may experience the condition differently. One common thread is that it can feel that the arthritis is happening to you, and that you have no control. But this is not the case. With the tools in this book, you have the means to make a difference to your mental and physical wellbeing – no matter how big or how small.

With lifestyle changes and lifestyle medicine, there is the potential to reduce your symptoms alongside your medication. One patient who had rheumatoid arthritis completely cut their dairy intake and saw an improvement while on medication, before trying a wholefood plant-based diet that led to them stopping medication completely. And a psoriatic arthritis patient saw their psoriasis and arthritic symptoms improve on a wholefood plant-based diet. These are just two examples, and while not everyone may want to go fully plant based (fatty fish, for instance, has vital anti-inflammatory properties), cutting down on highly inflammatory processed foods will help.

Food is not the only anti-inflammatory component in this book; nutrition, sleep, exercise and emotional wellbeing all play a role too. And in order to decrease inflammation we need to work on these factors, which are the foundations of *Beat Arthritis Naturally* and intertwined in Arthritis Foodie, by Emily.

Bringing this book into the world is the realisation of Emily's purpose behind Arthritis Foodie: to help people living with arthritis to feel better – with their arthritis and about having their arthritis. The book joins together Emily's personal experience of arthritis, scientific research and expert advice to fulfil her mission for the world to beat arthritis naturally.

Dr Micah Yu
Integrative rheumatologist at Dr Lifestyle,
Orange County, California

Introduction

You, your body and your life are at the mercy of your arthritis, and it has the control. But starting from today, it is time for you to take that control back. Rather than, 'I suffer with arthritis', say, 'I live with arthritis'. Say it out loud: I live with arthritis. It is a part of your life; you live with it and you can learn to live alongside it – you can beat arthritis by taking control. You can *live* with arthritis, *talk* about it and *feel better* in your body and mind by understanding it, and doing something about it. You are at step one already, reading this book. You are willing to transform your life by living with your arthritis in a new way.

There are, in fact, 100 types of arthritis and musculoskeletal conditions, affecting an estimated 350 million people globally. And many of those who are living with a form of arthritis are under 35 years old. Yet when you say the word 'arthritis', more often than not, people conjure up the stereotype of somebody elderly.

Arthritis can happen to anyone at any age, whether they are a 4-year-old, a teenager, a young adult or a grandparent. If you are not elderly when you notice the first signs or symptoms of arthritis, it can be hard to recognise – even for your GP – because of a widespread lack of awareness and understanding of the condition. And it is not just creaky joints either, with symptoms such as joint pain and swelling, stiffness, difficulty or restriction of movement, fatigue and poor sleep.

Living with pain is not easy. There are good days and bad days, but every day the arthritis is there. Currently, there is no cure for arthritis, and it can leave you feeling helpless, depressed and far from in control of your own body. The intention of this book is to enable you to take action. It's your chance to control your attitude towards your body and how you treat it – because who is living inside of it? Nobody but you. You are the one to make it a better place to live in, and to live with your arthritis.

Think about it this way. If you have to live with someone every day, 365 days, 24 hours, 1,440 minutes and 86,400 seconds of the day, actively and angrily wishing that person would leave is fine up to a point, but *mentally exhausting* if you do it every day. Isn't it easier to be friends with them than to make them an enemy? Isn't it easier to try to understand them than to ignore them? Isn't it better to make life with them the best it can possibly be? Making peace with your condition and learning everything you can to live better with it – beating it naturally – is about taking control of your body and your mindset. Your arthritis is not about to miraculously disappear – there is no magic potion, superfood smoothie or overnight therapy – but with the many strands of health and lifestyle improvements and advice in these pages, it can get quieter.

Will Lifestyle and Food Cure My Arthritis?

The short and truthful answer is no – not on their own. There is no evidence that they will cure the disease; so far, they have not cured mine – but what they have done is help me to manage my symptoms and live more healthily and happily alongside it.

As 'Plant Power Doctor' Dr Gemma Newman says:

> Arthritis has a common denominator, inflammation, so taking the time to naturally reduce your inflammatory markers is a way to relieve your symptoms and manage your condition. Eating anti-inflammatory foods, with a healthful plant-based diet, can be done alongside any treatment you may be receiving from your rheumatologist and should not be thought of as a replacement, but rather an augmentation of medical therapy from which to reduce need for medications if possible.

Exercise is anti-inflammatory, and it too is essential – even when you have an active disease, as you will see in Chapter 7. Add a lack of movement to poor diet and you have a recipe for being overweight, resulting in more inflammation and even less enthusiasm for physical activity. A decline in mental health can also often be a symptom of living with a chronic condition (who wouldn't struggle mentally when waking up in pain every day?) and new research has discovered a direct connection between depression and inflammation (see Chapter 9). The pain of the condition (see Chapter 6), plus the snooze-inducing-medication, general fatigue and lack of sleep really are *exhausting* (see Chapter 8). And food influences mood too, as both your brain and immune health are derived from your gut. It's evident that we must be mindful of what we eat (see Chapters 2–5) and how we look after ourselves in the long term.

Who has contributed to this book?

The book draws content from leading researchers, doctors and experts, and has had direct support in certain areas from the following contributors:

- Dr Micah Yu, Integrative Rheumatologist at Dr Lifestyle, Orange County, California
- Victoria Jain, 'The Autoimmunity Nutritionist', Pilates instructor, BSc in biochemistry with immunology
- Professor Paul Emery OBE, Versus Arthritis, Professor of Rheumatology and Director of the NIHR Leeds Biomedical Research Centre
- Dr Lauren Freid, Rheumatologist Clinical Instructor of Medicine, UCLA
- Steve Haines, chiropractor and author
- Zoe McKenzie, 'Actively Autoimmune', physiotherapist, personal trainer, gym and Pilates instructor
- Dr Jenna Macciochi, immunologist, author of *Immunity*, lecturer at University of Sussex
- Dr Gemma Newman, 'Plant Power Doctor', author and GP
- Dr Rupy Aujla, 'The Doctor's Kitchen', author and GP
- Raj Vara, pharmacist for over 40 years, superintendent pharmacist at Husbands Pharmacy, one of the oldest in London

What About Scientific Research?

Where there is research available, I have deciphered it and worked it into something more digestible. Despite a large proportion of this leaning towards RA, OA, PsA, AIDs (autoimmune diseases) and chronic inflammation, I have tried to achieve a balanced view on the condition and how we can all live better alongside it. For references, please see p. 269.

Will I Need to Remove Any Food Categories From My Diet?

With food, there is no one-size-fits-all, and where some people may find they react negatively to a particular substance, others may not. Rheumatologist Lauren Freid encourages patients to become interested in diet and to be as informed as they can be about anti-inflammatory and pro-inflammatory foods (more on these later) – she also advocates for a wholefood, plant-predominant diet, with an avoidance of processed foods.

It's also important to remember, though, that food is the foundation for many social interactions, which support emotional and mental wellbeing. It is essential to learn how to eat for your body and your arthritis, so that you can continue to enjoy food and allow it to bring you together with others. Celebrity personal trainer Nicola Addison explains that an 80/20 rule is a helpful approach, meaning that we make healthy choices 80 per cent of the time (accepting that we cannot always be perfect) regarding exercise, sleep, managing stress and alcohol intake.

So, never feel guilty for wanting to enjoy a moment with family or friends, at Christmas or on social occasions. Tracking if or when you notice changes is important, to be able to be mindful of the effects in the future (more on this in Chapter 4), but I must emphasise that this is personal. You know your body better than anyone else.

Should I Consult My GP or Specialist Before Implementing Changes?

Beat Arthritis Naturally is simply about taking back control of your health through natural means, but if you have any concerns about the contents of this book and you are unsure as to how it may impact any underlying health conditions that you have, please consult your medical professional – either your GP or specialist (a rheumatologist, for example). This book is by no means a replacement for your current therapy, so please do not stop taking your prescribed medications unless advised to do so by your medical specialist.

*

With the support of expert advice from leading researchers, doctors, rheumatologists, immunologists, nutritionists, physiotherapists, pharmacists and other health experts, *Beat Arthritis Naturally* will give you the confidence you need to live a healthier and happier life. This book is your time to listen, learn and absorb a new approach to managing and living with arthritis – find all the time you need to take it in.

This is not a book you read once, then leave on the shelf.

This is not a book you use as a doorstop or decoration.

This is not a book you forget about.

Beat Arthritis Naturally is the book you read over and over again. It's the book that gets a little messy with every recipe you make; the book you dip into before bed to remind yourself of an exercise sequence, pain relief or sleep remedy. It is your map, your manual and your motivation. Turn down the page corners, sticky-note your favourite parts, scribble and highlight the sentences you will return to. Love – and learn from – this book: it will be with you on your journey to living better with arthritis, every step of the way.

1
All About Arthritis

'Anything that's human is mentionable, and anything that is mentionable can be more manageable.'
Fred McFeely Rogers, American TV host and producer

How did I end up here, writing this book for you? Perhaps it would be a good starting point for you to know a bit about Arthritis Foodie.

Your genetics hold the bullets in the gun, but your environment pulls the trigger. My environment was a friend's barbeque, summer 2013. I was run-down, having taught in Italy as a tutor for six weeks without a break, and my immune system was crying out for rest, vitamins, hydration and good gut bugs. Instead, what I gave it was exhaustion, dehydration in the form of alcohol and food poisoning. While I am not completely certain that I can pinpoint the demise of my immune system to this particular day, it had previously had one blip when I was 4 years old and I was hospitalised for a week with swollen knees. That was definitely the start of living with arthritis.

Eating and drinking whatever I pleased from that barbeque buffet – including processed meats and starchy white bread – I bit into food poisoning that lasted over a fortnight. Shortly after, my ring finger on my right hand swelled up like a balloon on the verge of popping (which I now know was dactylitis – see p. 18). As I returned to university for my final year, more than one finger began to swell and my thumbs too. My skin was so painful to touch and I could not sleep (or talk) for sneezing. These symptoms remained for months, becoming progressively worse, but I explained them away as 'a bit of hay fever', 'a cold' or 'freshers' flu'.

But I was in a state of chronic inflammation and – although I didn't know it at the time – it was an autoimmune disease. The thing with autoimmune diseases is that they are not easily explained with a quick diagnosis, speedy recovery, easy medicinal solution and *voila*! You are better. Rather, they are drawn-out processes, affecting mind and body, as you are dragged through consultation rooms, hospital corridors and departments, prescribed a myriad painkillers and medications, probed, poked and prodded like a pincushion. Sitting in hospital waiting rooms becomes normality. And since starting the Arthritis Foodie community and speaking with so many of you, it is clear to me that there is rarely a fast diagnosis or a treatment that works straight away.

Eventually, I was sent to a rheumatologist who, at the time, proposed that the pain was 'all in my head', which I now understand to be a form of medical gaslighting: a healthcare professional downplays or denies the symptoms you know you are experiencing, and instead tries to convince you that they are caused by something else, or that you are imagining them. Over the course of two years, my diagnosis went from fibromyalgia to reactive arthritis, before finally – and permanently – landing on 'seronegative arthritis', described as being in between rheumatoid arthritis and psoriatic arthritis. I tried all kinds of medications – steroid injections, naproxen, sulfasalazine – all with little to no effect. By Christmas 2015, after four months of gradually increasing the dosage, I was taking 20mg of methotrexate (an immunosuppressant drug) weekly, 5mg of folic acid five times a week (to help protect the healthy cells in my body) and having biweekly blood tests to monitor my liver function.

But my arthritis was *not me*; it was *separate from* me. It felt like a squatter was living in my home, causing damp and cracks in the walls, spoiling what I thought my life should 'look like' and 'be like' as a young person. So, I hid it. I painted over the damp and plastered over the cracks. I hid it from everyone and even tried to hide it from myself. Desperate to be 'normal' – and by 'normal', I mean *my* normal and living like I would have done before my arthritis – I pushed myself and my body to its limits, even when I knew I would suffer for it. And *believe me*, I always suffered for trying to keep up, frequently ill with flu-like symptoms. Regularly, I would still go into work when I should have been in bed because I was so worried about losing my job, or being judged, or being seen as incapable compared to my picture-of-health colleagues.

When taking methotrexate, your alcohol consumption is limited to the national guideline recommendations of 14 units spread out during the week, but at 22, I felt the unspoken social pressure to 'join in'. I became accustomed to pouring drinks away or 'losing them'. I confided in a friend about my condition and he would discreetly drink them for me. It was amusing to see him become more inebriated than he had intended to be, until I started to get some of the blame for his hangovers. Now I no longer feel the pressure to drink, so I don't, and I am happy to say why, but it has taken time to get here. Never apologise to people, society or the world for doing what is right for you.

The swelling in my hands began to reduce and the pain subsided too, but when you have arthritis, you cannot ever sit back, relax and think that it has gone. You know that's not possible, so the thought of it lingers in the back of your mind. *Still there underneath the wallpaper. Will it worsen in my hands again? What if it flares up somewhere else? My knee again, or my feet? What if I can't walk?* During a period of remission, all of these thoughts whisper in the background, but despite them, you make the most out of feeling your 'normal', because you do not know how long it will last.

Despite the improvement, I was still fatigued and I did feel poorly regularly. My lifestyle, eating habits and job did not help. My mum would always say to me, 'Emily, please stop burning the candle at both ends'. Working or socialising in the evenings, often until late, I grabbed sandwiches or foods requiring minimal preparation, like pasta or fish fingers. My diet included processed or preserved foods, refined carbohydrates, sugar-filled sauces and cakes, and I pushed the boundaries on caffeine and alcohol. We only get one body to take care of, so we must do all that we can to do that well, but at this point in time I was not taking much care of mine at all. And I had zero awareness of what my body needed in terms of rest, exercise or mental wellbeing either.

During Christmas 2017, I had a nasty flu, and could not remember being so poorly since the arthritis first began in 2013. Hot and cold sweats, sleepless nights, headaches, blocked sinuses, fatigue, my entire body aching, coughing and sneezing, and – a strange signal for me – white spots on my tongue. My body was having a complete meltdown. My heart sank. My symptoms lasted for more than three weeks. I felt powerless. Then, just as I started to feel better, I looked down and saw the start of a lump in my right ankle, and that all-too-familiar stiff, fluid-like feeling.

My rheumatologist's solution, as an interim measure while waiting for an available appointment, was to have a steroid injection in my gluteus maximus muscle, aka *derrière*, and to increase my methotrexate dosage, with a review after three months. I thought, *Great, the medication will sort it out, it's out of my control.* I began wearing ankle supports, icing or heating my ankle at night and taking strong painkillers. That steroid injection kept my pain at bay for a few months, but the next one had no effect, and the increase in methotrexate did not help either.

Still, I would tell myself: *Nobody can tell I am in pain. Nobody knows the extent of my pain. Nobody wants or needs to know. Nobody my age has arthritis. Nobody sees my arthritis. Nobody sees my pain. Just keep going . . .*

But it got worse. Out with my mum and sister, I was in so much agony that I had to sit on benches outside while they shopped. Similarly, on holiday with my friends, the pain was so sickening and unbearable one day that I had to sit on a chair in the supermarket while they grabbed our groceries. Most days, I would try so hard to hide it, and it was an exhausting mental burden. I do not do this now.

Joint swelling in arthritis can mirror from one side of the body to the other. By the summer of 2018, I had swelling in both of my ankles and in my leg above my right ankle. When I was away with friends, I woke up with another new flare one morning. My right arm, elbow and shoulder felt peculiar and painful. I tried to stretch my arm, but physically couldn't. My elbow was so swollen it had literally bent my arm. I played it down and said I had just slept funny on it, but this became a real breaking point for me.

Completely disengaged from my body, I had given over control of it to the methotrexate. But it was time to take it back. I started to think about how I treated my own body. Could I help it – and the arthritis – through lifestyle changes? I bought a few arthritis food-based books that were extremely outdated, a range of healthy recipe books and logged on to social media, eager to find someone talking about living with arthritis and natural ways to beat it. But I just could not find what I was picturing. Where was the account dedicated to food and arthritis? A community, with people like me, where I could learn how to manage my symptoms naturally?

And then it clicked.

If it did not exist, if nobody else was doing it, then I would. And maybe I could help anyone else who was looking for it too . . . And that is how Arthritis Foodie began.

What is Arthritis? A Comprehensive Look

Living with arthritis can feel isolating, and the Arthritis Foodie community's mission is to make sure people do not feel alone. Because you aren't.

As mentioned earlier, arthritis and other joint-related conditions affect millions of people around the world and can happen to anyone at any age. For starters, here is a short list of celebrities who are living with a form of the condition:

- Lady Gaga (fibromyalgia)
- Andy Murray (osteoarthritis)
- Robbie Williams (arthritis – back)
- Kim Kardashian (psoriatic arthritis)
- Tiger Woods (osteoarthritis)
- Kristy McPherson (juvenile arthritis)
- Jo Whiley (rheumatoid arthritis)
- Tatum O'Neal (rheumatoid arthritis)
- Paddy McGuinness (rheumatoid arthritis)
- Laura Wright (juvenile arthritis)
- Liam Gallagher (arthritis – hips)

Worldwide, musculoskeletal disorders, which include all forms of arthritis, are ranked as the second-most common cause of disability. Arthritis exists in all races, age groups and sexes. As I've said, arthritis does not always equal old, and if we can continue to debunk this myth, it may enable those of us who have it to live more openly with our condition. The ramifications of this could be a reduction in the mental burden of the condition, which would, in turn, ease the physical one. *I hope*.

Types of arthritis

There are various conditions linked to joint pain and swelling, with osteoarthritis (OA) and rheumatoid arthritis (RA) known as the two most common types. Many are autoimmune diseases (AIDs), which are chronic inflammatory disorders caused by abnormal immune-system function that may be initiated by environmental factors, viruses, toxic chemicals or genetic factors. This immune-system abnormality is described as your body 'attacking itself': your immune system fails to recognise your body's own cells as 'self', or belonging to you, viewing them instead as a disease to be combatted – or mistaking friend for foe.

Studies have shown that around a third of all AIDs are genetically predisposed, while the remainder are due to environmental triggers, as well as diet, disturbances to the gut and digestive systems and other lifestyle factors. It's that gun, bullets and trigger analogy again. Whether immunity-based or not, arthritis is a chronic and painful condition without a cure. So the more we can understand it – and learn to manage a life with it – the lighter the affliction may feel.

ARTHRITIS AT A GLANCE

The following are the main types of arthritis:

- Osteoarthritis (OA)
- Rheumatoid arthritis (RA) [AID]
- Psoriatic arthritis (PsA) [AID]
- Juvenile idiopathic arthritis (JIA) [AID]
- Reactive arthritis (ReA) [AID]
- Ankylosing spondylitis (AS) [AID]
- Gout

Typical symptoms include:

- Joint pain, swelling and stiffness
- Difficultly and restriction in movement
- Fatigue and sleep disturbance
- Decline in mental wellbeing
- Muscle wasting

Osteoarthritis

OA is the most prevalent joint disease worldwide. It is a wear-and-tear condition in which physical deterioration in the cartilage and bones leads to pain, loss of joint function and disability. The knee is the most common site in the body for OA, followed by the hips, hands and wrists.

The onset of this condition is twofold: primary OA is associated with ageing (but is not caused by it), whereas secondary OA frequently appears earlier in life and is typically instigated by injury, a stressful job, diabetes or obesity. It is generally not included among inflammatory diseases, but increasingly evidence indicates that inflammation does play a central role in its development, induced by pro-inflammatory cytokines. Cytokines are a bit like WiFi – signalling molecules that enable communication between the cells of the immune system and other non-immune cells. We will come across these again throughout the book.

Rheumatoid arthritis (RA)

RA is the most prevalent inflammatory arthritis, associated with high levels of oxidative stress. Females are affected three times more than males. It is an autoimmune condition and characteristically it occurs in the same joints on both sides of the body, but there may also be inflammation of skin, eyes, heart or lungs. The exact origins of RA are believed to be multifaceted, and studies suggest that both environmental and genetic factors are at play, also noting the release of pro-inflammatory cytokines, as described above.

There are two forms: seropositive and seronegative (the one I have). Those with seropositive test positive in their bloodwork for the rheumatoid factor (RF) and/or anti-CCP (an antibody present in most RA patients), whereas those with the seronegative form test negatively for both. Other blood-monitoring terms that you may have come across are the C-reactive protein (CRP), or erythrocyte sedimentation rate (ESR), associated with acute and chronic inflammation, including infection, cancer and AIDs. Now that you know what these are, you may feel more comfortable discussing your levels of them with your rheumatologist, as I like to.

Psoriatic arthritis (PsA)

Closely related to RA, this is a type of spondyloarthritis (SpA), describing a group of inflammatory rheumatic diseases induced by a complex mixture of genetic, immunological and environmental factors. Unlike RA, however, PsA is experienced asymmetrically, is usually seronegative and affects tendons. PsA may also involve the skin condition psoriasis. Dactylitis is also a distinguishing feature of PsA, which is characterised by sausage-shaped swelling of the toes or fingers (a clear signal in my early experience).

Juvenile idiopathic arthritis (JIA)

In the UK alone, about 15,000 children are living with JIA. It is the most commonly diagnosed rheumatic condition in children, but JIA is not a disease – it is a collective term, with a set of diagnostics that includes symptoms of arthritis forming before a child's 16th birthday, lasting for at least six weeks and with an unknown origin. The word 'idiopathic' relates to any disease or condition that develops unexpectedly and has an undetermined cause.

JIA conditions seem to be the childhood equivalent of those observed in adults, and at least one third of children with JIA will continue to have an active form of arthritis in adulthood. My suspicion is that my 'idiopathic' swollen knees that lasted a week when I was a child were the early signs of inflammatory arthritis.

Reactive arthritis (ReA)

ReA is inflammation in one or multiple joints caused by an infection within the body. The infection may derive from the gut, urinary tract or reproductive organs. Reiter's syndrome – a triad of arthritis, urethritis and conjunctivitis – is a common example of ReA. ReA symptoms usually develop around one to three weeks after exposure to the cause of the infection. Bacteria and bugs that are often responsible for causing ReA are chlamydia, yersinia, salmonella, shigella and campylobacter.

ReA can also be associated with auto-inflammatory or immunologic disorders such as Crohn's disease, ulcerative colitis, rheumatic conditions and hereditary auto-inflammatory disorders. For most people, ReA disappears completely within six months, but in 10 to 20 per cent of cases, the symptoms last for longer. In some situations, people may go on to develop an ongoing type of arthritis that requires long-term treatment.

Ankylosing spondylitis (AS)

AS is an AID and seronegative inflammatory condition that largely affects the spine and pelvis. The average age of onset for AS is 24, and it is generally associated with an inflammation of the spinal joints and surrounding structures, resulting in pain, stiffness and limitation of movement. Pain and stiffness of the limb-based joints, including the hips and shoulders, are also present in around a third of patients with AS. Treatment usually involves physiotherapy and anti-inflammatory drugs.

Gout

Gout (also known as monosodium urate crystal deposition disease) is a type of inflammatory arthritis, and a hereditary metabolic disorder. An abnormal build-up of monosodium urate crystals in and around the joints features in episodes of acute arthritis, caused by having too much of the chemical uric acid in the bloodstream. The most prevalent cause of inflammatory arthritis in men aged over 50, gout affects 1–2 per cent of adult men in the Western world, and is far more common in males than females. It was first identified as early as 2640 BC, by the ancient Egyptians.

In gout, the uric-acid crystals can also deposit in tendons, kidneys and other tissues, as well as the joints, causing inflammation and damage.

FIBROMYALGIA AND LUPUS

Fibromyalgia and lupus are two widespread conditions which, while not technically counted as arthritis, are commonly associated with it.

Fibromyalgia

Fibromyalgia is a chronic-pain-syndrome with an unknown cause. It involves a wide spectrum of symptoms such as allodynia (pain from stimuli that do not normally cause pain, such as lightly touching your skin), debilitating fatigue, joint stiffness and migraines. Fibromyalgia is also accompanied by sleep disturbances, cognitive dysfunction, anxiety or depressive episodes.

There are still many physicians who refuse to believe that fibromyalgia exists, assuming that a patient's pain is 'all in their head'. Although it is not classified as an AID, it can often manifest with one – such as RA, for example. A multidisciplinary approach to treatment involving both pharmacological and non-pharmacological interventions is advised.

Lupus

Lupus is an AID that is roughly around nine times more common in women than men. There are two main types of lupus: discoid lupus and systemic lupus ery-thematosus (SLE). Discoid lupus only affects the skin, causing rashes in widespread or small areas of the body, whereas SLE lupus – like RA – can affect many different parts of the body, and most people will have one or a few of the possible symptoms (such as joint pain, skin rashes, fatigue, fever, weight loss, swelling of the lymph glands) and these will ebb and flow. More common in younger people, the precise cause is not yet known, but it is evident that both genetic predisposition and environmental triggers are factors.

Current therapies for arthritis

Mainstream treatments consist of medication, physiotherapy and surgery, depending on the type of arthritis that you have and its severity.

Medicinal therapies

There are numerous medicinal treatments given, dependent upon your arthritis severity, but typically a patient will begin on one, before trying the next (the try, test and trial period is 12 weeks to see if it helps). You may be prescribed one or a combination of drugs, and this can be temporary, for short-term relief, or ongoing, for long-term management of your condition.

- **Disease-modifying anti-rheumatic drugs** (DMARDs) are usually the first stop and include:
    - sulfasalazine
    - hydroxychloroquine
    - methotrexate
    - leflunomide
- **Biological treatments** such as etanercept and infliximab are frequently taken in combination with a DMARD, such as methotrexate. These tend to be used only if DMARDs alone have not been effective.
- **JAK inhibitors**, including tofacitinib and baricitinib, were introduced in 2012 for those with severe RA who have not found DMARDs or biologics effective.
- **Non-steroidal anti-inflammatory drugs** (NSAIDs) can help to relieve pain while also reducing inflammation, but it is worth noting that long-term use may accelerate OA:
    - ibuprofen
    - naproxen
    - diclofenac
    - celecoxib
    - etoricoxib

- **Steroids** – usually (but not always) in the form of an injection, either directly into a painful joint or into a muscle to help multiple joints. They are generally given to provide short-term pain relief while waiting for other medication or struggling mid-flare.
- **Painkillers** – although they do not treat the inflammation in your joints, these may be helpful in relieving pain and include paracetamol, codeine or co-codamol.
- **Capsaicin cream** – a topical pain reliever that works by blocking the nerves that send pain messages in the treated area (more on this in Chapter 6).

Physiotherapy

One of the pillars of mainstream therapy for arthritis, physiotherapy is looked at in much more detail on pp. 185–188 (along with chiropractic and osteopathy, as well as rehabilitative care, such as occupational therapy and podiatry).

Surgery

If a joint has been severely altered by arthritis, surgery may improve mobility and quality of life. Generally, it is only needed in a small number of patients where other treatments have not been effective or more support is required. Types of surgery include:

- joint replacement – such as for the hip, knee or shoulder joints
- joint fusing – where a joint replacement is not suitable,

a surgeon may suggest an operation to fuse a joint in a permanent position
- osteotomy – in those with osteoarthritis in the knees who are not suitable for knee-replacement surgery this can help to realign the knee and readjust the weight upon it
- finger, hand and wrist surgery – such as carpal-tunnel release
- arthroscopy – a procedure to remove inflamed joint tissue

The Foundations of Beating Arthritis Naturally

Because there are various types of arthritis, and taking into account age, environment and genetics, the condition manifests differently from one person to the next. But, as previously mentioned, several lifestyle factors – including diet, exercise, sleep and emotional well-being – can have an impact.

According to professor of rheumatology Paul Emery:

> '. . . exercise, sleeping well, eating healthily – for example, the Mediterranean Diet (MD), all of which help in managing chronic autoimmune/arthritic/inflammatory conditions, alongside medication. The MD has even been useful in showing that it reduces pain mediators, but nobody has shown whether or not it can prevent arthritis, as yet. There is evidence to say that the bowel is abnormal in patients with arthritis. The argument is whether or not you can change it, and if you stop your intervention whether or not it [the bowel] just returns to the way it was before, but if you maintain on the right diet there is no reason why the improvement couldn't be maintained.'

And Dr Lauren Freid comments: 'If you're taking a medicine with the purpose of fighting inflammation and reducing pain, why wouldn't you also take the lifestyle approaches to achieve the same effect? Medicine will only go so far if lifestyle continues to drive inflammation that will counteract its effects.'

It may feel overwhelming at first, but this book is your starting point. It is your set of stepping stones, and every chapter is a step in the right direction. In the words of writer and illustrator Charlie Mackesy, 'One of our greatest freedoms is how we react to things'. In other words, managing how you feel and think about having arthritis, as well as how you react to it, are key to being able to advance changes in both your body and your mind. The tools in this book will facilitate this holistic approach.

Befriend your gut

The gut is the main protagonist in this story. Pretty much everything we ever feel is associated with our gut microbiome – in fact, the gut houses almost 70 per cent of our entire immune system, and produces hormones that influence anything from appetite to mood. So we should be feeding and fuelling our gut bugs properly.

What exactly is the gut microbiome, you might ask? Well, it is an immense ecosystem of organisms and microbes such as bacteria, yeasts, fungi and viruses that live in our digestive systems. *And what is the difference between the gut microbiome and the gut microbiota?* Often used interchangeably, microbiota is the actual bugs (microorganism), whereas microbiome refers to the bugs *and* their genes (there's actually a staggering 22 million bacterial genes in the gut microbiome).

Collectively, the gut microbiome is heavier than the average brain, weighing up to 2 kilograms, and it is increasingly becoming established as an organ in its own right, research showing that we are likely to be around 50:50 human and microbes. Each gut contains about 100 trillion vital bacteria that break down food and toxins, make vitamins and influence our immune system. The immune system, much like the gut microbiome, is not one place or one thing, but a collection of things in a number of places. As articulated by immunologist Dr Jenna Macciochi, immunity is a fusion of leukocytes (white blood cells), lymphatic organs, cytokines (signalling molecules) and their combined mixture of biological functions.

Not only is the gut heavier than the average brain, it actually *contains* a very thin layer of brain. BBC's Dr Michael Mosley writes in astonishment that this layer of brain (called the enteric system) is made up of the same cells (neurons) that are found in the brain *and* there are over 100 million of them in the gut – the same number you would find in the brain of a cat. (Yes! I managed to get a cat into this book, and yes, I will look at Molly, my cat, a little differently now.)

With the gut being a pivotal part of our health and wellbeing, it is not, then, a wild revelation that an unhappy gut equals an afflicted body and mind. Research is uncovering connections between gut health and disease manifestation, both mental and physical. Depression often accompanies many of these diseases, including arthritis, psoriasis, multiple sclerosis (MS), irritable bowel syndrome (IBS), inflammatory bowel disease (IBD), autism, Alzheimer's and many more.

Many doctors feel that their training is sorely lacking when it comes to nutrition. If my doctor had been sufficiently trained in gut health and nutrition, could this have led to a quicker diagnosis or a more suitable treatment? Non-profit organisation Culinary Medicine UK (CMUK), led by Dr Rupy Aujla, has taken its lead from the Goldring Centre for Culinary Medicine (GCCM) in the USA, and developed a programme to teach doctors and medical students in the UK the foundations of nutrition – from the practical aspects of cooking, to the science of food and its application in clinical practice.

Whether your doctor has grasped the importance of nutrition or not, ensuring that your gut is happy is essential, so this includes feeding your gut microbiota with the ultimate diet, including the phytochemicals (see Chapter 2) that are being studied by scientists as additional therapies for obesity and inflammatory diseases. Good nutrition can provide and preserve good health; conversely, poor nutrition can increase the risk of developing chronic degenerative diseases. Our eating habits influence all aspects of our biology, from our metabolisms to our immune systems to our guts. But the response that we receive from diet is individual and depends on everything from genetics to our guts, sex and immune systems.

As mentioned, a good place to start is the MD, typically consisting of a high intake of vegetables, fruits, nuts, legumes and extra virgin olive oil, with moderate intakes of fish, poultry meat and dairy products, less red meat and a moderate amount of red wine. It has been shown to preserve human health in a myriad of ways, from protecting against cancer and cardiovascular disease to preventing alterations in gut microbiota composition and the subsequent inflammation, exerting long term anti-inflammatory effects. The MD is definitely a foundation for the recipe ideas in this book.

But let's get back to arthritis again because, funnily enough, scientists suspected an interaction between the gut and arthritis decades before the more recent exploration and interest in the gut microbiome. In fact, Professor Emery notes that the UK's largest arthritis charity, Versus Arthritis, has been researching this connection, with microbiologists posing the question: 'Do gut bacteria play a role in rheumatoid arthritis?' An animal study demonstrated the role of the gut microbiome in modulating arthritis progression and multiple studies have demonstrated dysbiosis (impaired and imbalanced gut) in RA patients. And some researchers have suggested that genetic factors alone do not appear to be sufficient to develop the disease, stating that an environmental trigger, such as variations in our microbiome, is likely to be required to initiate inflammatory arthritis in individuals with a genetic predisposition.

Immunologist Dan Littman of New York University has taken it one step further and speculated that RA in humans might also be due to *specific* gut microbes through a study involving a group of 114 residents within the New York City area – some healthy, others living with treated RA, some PsA and others with new and recently diagnosed RA, who were not yet receiving treatment. In the newly diagnosed, a bacterium named *Prevotella copri* was present in 75 per cent of patients' intestines, whereas it only appeared in 37 per cent of those living with either RA or PsA and just 21 per cent of healthy individuals.

Undeniably, more research is needed to explore the association between diet and the gut microbiome and how this can influence RA pathogenesis, or even other forms of inflammatory, immune-related chronic diseases. As diet can influence the gut microbiome, perhaps diseases can be manipulated through diet and alteration of gut bacteria, but research is still in its infancy. Who knows, in 20 years' time, I could be revisiting this book with some amendments . . . But, in the meantime, we know that there's plenty we can be doing.

Be mindful of your body

The gut has plenty to answer for. It is our second brain, after all. But there's lots that goes on outside of it when you are burdened with a chronic disease paired with chronic inflammation. Anything from stress to a poor night's sleep, to a nutrition-less meal, to sitting down all day can lead to an excess of inflammation. Being aware and present around how your body is feeling, both mentally and physically – taking the steps to understand your pain, your body and your brain a little better – is also an underpinning principle and foundation of this book.

*

Your arthritis, body, and genetics belong to you – your experience of this condition may look entirely different to mine, or you may have found some strands of my story in yours. Either way, I hope that you are now beginning to feel emboldened as you begin to learn more about managing your arthritis using the tools in this book as part of a holistic approach.

2

Anti-Inflammatory Essentials

'One cannot think well, love well, sleep well, if one has not dined well.'
Virginia Woolf, author

Aloe vera on sunburn? Tea tree oil for an acne breakout? Vinegar-soaked bandage for a wound? Do any of these sound relatable, or were my family's natural methods a little off the wall? I'm going to hazard a guess that you have some similar stories of natural remedies being used in your home, or by your grandparents. The therapeutic use of plants and their natural by-products is as ancient as human civilisation, and a study conducted by the World Health Organization (WHO) reported that even now, about 80 per cent of the world's population relies on traditional medicine.

For centuries, plants provided the primary source for drugs, and around a quarter of medicines prescribed globally still come from them. But no, I am not about to tell you to throw away your medication for a herbal tea – *don't* do that. It is worth noting though that since the new millennium we have begun to go back to our roots, reassessing natural products as a source of bioactive compounds for the treatment of numerous conditions.

Food is one brushstroke on the colourful canvas of our health: our immune system, gut microbiome, physical and mental health are all influenced by our environment and how we take care of our bodies, including what we put into them, so food is a good place to begin. Driven to discover how we can live better with arthritis, I have researched the subject extensively, looking into key anti-inflammatory foods, vitamins and minerals, an assortment of spices, the Mediterranean diet (MD), Ayurvedic medicine and Chinese medicine. If it's out there, *I've explored it*.

If you are already a follower of Arthritis Foodie, you will have seen that I've spent numerous weekends with my head in books or scouring digital resources at the British Library. I'm very thorough! So, with the knowledge gleaned from books, articles and papers, this chapter (and those that follow) will examine it all. And if you would like to investigate further yourself, my references are also listed at the end of the book (see p. 269).

Getting into Genetics

Once thought of as anecdotal, historically embedded expressions such as, 'You are what you eat' or, 'Food is medicine' (derived from Hippocrates' philosophy in 400 BC), arguably now hold *some* scientific weight. The University of Oxford unveiled genetic evidence that our diets can affect the DNA sequences of our genes on a generational timescale, proving that by adopting different diets we can actually alter our genetic make-up.

But before you start wondering if a piece of broccoli will give you a new and improved knee joint, let me be clear: we cannot tear up and throw away the DNA blueprint we were handed at birth and replace it with a new one. We *can*, however, manipulate our health for the better now and for any future offspring.

On the topic of genetics, it is vital to note that the health studies I have drawn from in this book are generally populated with, and written by, white males, with little or no diversity. Unpicking the systemic racism and inequality in science is too hefty a topic for me to explore in this book, but I urge you to educate yourself further and to be mindful of this throughout.

The Gut, Food and Inflammation: A Unique Mystery

Research into the gut microbiome is developing by the minute, and there is so much we are still learning about the immune system too. Everyone's body, gut, immune system and arthritis are different – because *we* are all different. Sounds obvious, doesn't it? But it's why research results may not always be tangible when it comes to humans and why, therefore, there is a scarcity of human clinical evidence in relation to food.

It's in our DNA

Plants contain an array of micronutrients, vitamins, minerals and phytonutrients (or phytochemicals). Food has the ability to interact with our DNA, and alongside other lifestyle factors (see Chapters 7, 8 and 9) it has the potential to change the expression of our genes – described as nutrigenetics. As mentioned, our genes go unchanged, but we can alter their output (how they behave within us) with the input they receive (from our food or environmental factors).

Can food really fight inflammation?

Because inflammation is one of the most common denominators in people living with arthritis, I have focused here on nutritional compounds that have been scientifically linked to reducing inflammation, and/or having anti-arthritic effects.

There are a number of plant-based compounds that are thought to help keep our inflammation and inflammatory responses in check. But, in truth, it's a lot more diverse and complex than simply taking a shot of turmeric and ginger juice – although I do enjoy doing that too. And, to reiterate, this research is still in its very early stages – what we have uncovered so far is a mere fragment of the whole.

Pure Plants = Phytonutrients

We have all come across the fundamental nutrients that get all the airtime, i.e. proteins, minerals and vitamins. But besides these, there are naturally occurring and powerful bioactive compounds known as phytonutrients, and there are more than 25,000 of them around – from carotenoid to polyphenol, probiotic to prebiotic – found largely in plants, whether from the humble fruit or vegetable or the flavoursome herb or spice. Phytonutrients maintain and modulate immune function to prevent specific diseases, alongside having the potential to treat them – so, *naturally*, these all-natural products hold great promise in clinical therapy (like helping the symptoms of our arthritis).

The largest group of phytonutrients are polyphenols. At the time of writing, 8,000 types of polyphenols have been identified and they have probably existed in the plant kingdom for over 1 billion years. These incredible compounds are antioxidant (fighting inflammatory by-products called free radicals), anti-inflammatory, cardioprotective (RA heart health is paramount) and antimicrobial (fighting against harmful microorganisms). Polyphenols have a huge impact on our human cells, interacting with the essence of who we are – our DNA.

More and more studies strongly suggest that long-term consumption of diets rich in plant phytonutrients, like polyphenols, offer protection against the development of several chronic human illnesses and diseases.

Which ones matter to us?

Phytonutrients epigallocatechin gallate (EGCG), carnosol, hydroxytyrosol, curcumin, resveratrol, kaempferol and genistein have been the most widely examined in arthritis. And, although they sound like substances from another dimension, *trust me,* they really can be found on your plate or in a cup of tea. Typically, they're most beneficial when consumed in their natural whole form; so, curcumin supplements may not be as healthful as pure turmeric, for example.

How can I include them in my diet?

Try making changes – like green tea instead of coffee, homemade salad dressings with extra virgin olive oil instead of shop-bought ones or dark chocolate packed with antioxidants instead of the sugar-filled, processed, dairy version. These are just a few things you can do quite easily – and this book is your springboard. Below is a detailed overview of the science behind the compounds, but you can skip to the end of the chapter for an at-a-glance guide.

Green tea (epigallocatechin gallate – EGCG)

Globally, tea is the most consumed beverage after water. I think I probably drink more Yorkshire brews (made with black tea) than I do water. Yet green tea contains six times more polyphenols (such as EGCG) than black tea, while matcha has a staggering 137 times more antioxidants than green tea, with one cup being equivalent to ten cups of green tea. EGCG has been shown in some studies to alleviate inflammation and arthritis. I am probably 90 per cent made up of matcha green tea, as I drink it so frequently. But how much *should* you drink? It's fair to say that one cup a day should suffice, as green tea does contain caffeine, albeit a lot less than coffee. Get the kettle on!

Turmeric (curcumin)

Have any of you been told to try turmeric for your arthritis? (*Eye roll*) Now, a turmeric latte isn't going to provide much curcumin (the chief polyphenol found in turmeric), but turmeric remedies are not as out-there as you may think. Ten times more active as an antioxidant than vitamin E, exceeding the anti-arthritic activity of an NSAID, curcumin has shown some promising effects in patients with various pro-inflammatory diseases, including arthritis, irritable bowel disease (IBS) and psoriasis. Turmeric supplements, lattes, oil, powder, 'shots', topical creams . . . The list is endless, but what is best? Well, when digested alone, curcumin has poor absorption but piperine (found in black pepper) has been shown to increase absorption by 2,000 per cent. Piperine even has anti-inflammatory activity itself, so, don't forget to add it to the mix.

Ginger (gingerol)

Ginger is well established in traditional, Ayurvedic and Chinese medicine to alleviate nausea and pain. It's even been found to share pharmacological properties with NSAIDs. Gingerols in studies have been shown to protect against OA, RA and gout, defending bone cartilage from damage, suppressing joint swelling, preventing joint inflammation and destruction, lessening pain, reducing potent pro-inflammatory cytokines, decreasing the manifestations of disease and the severity of symptoms. Try throwing slices of fresh ginger into your stir-fry or adding ground ginger powder to a smoothie.

Extra virgin olive oil (hydroxytyrosol)

The glug-glug-glug of glorious extra virgin olive oil (EVOO) has become a daily feature in my cooking. Whether for roasting or drizzling, it's a deserving store-cupboard staple. Hydroxytyrosol is the most widely examined polyphenol in EVOO, acknowledged by both the U.S. Food and Drug Administration (FDA) and the European Food Safety Authority (EFSA) as something we should be getting every day. The latter recommends a daily consumption of 5mg hydroxytyrosol and its derivatives (so around 20g or 2 tablespoons of EVOO daily). EVOO has been shown to have positive effects on arthritis in terms of pain, inflammation and disease onset. Varying studies also indicate that EVOO may improve symptoms in chronic inflammatory and AIDs such as RA and psoriasis, but further research is needed. Avoid lower-quality olive oils (refined) if you can, as they lose antioxidant and anti-inflammatory capacities through overprocessing. Pure traditional extra virgin olive oil from little Italian village markets, hand-bottled by their makers, is like nothing else (believe me!).

Cinnamon (cinnamaldehyde)

My earliest memory of cinnamon is of my Nanan's homemade baked apple pie, which was oozing with it. Naturally, then, I associate the spice with sweet things, and its name, in fact, derives from a Greek word meaning 'sweet wood'. But I have also found it blends just as well with savoury foods, from curries to chutneys. It's one of the oldest traditional Ayurvedic medicines for inflammatory and pain-related conditions, its active polyphenolic component being cinnamaldehyde. In a range of studies, it has reduced inflammation by inhibiting inflammatory cytokines and reducing the tender and swollen joints count.

Some other polyphenols worthy of a quick mention

- **Carnosol:** carnosol is a major component of the culinary herbs sage, rosemary, thyme, marjoram, basil and oregano. Sage has been used for the treatment of gout, rheumatism and inflammation, while rosemary has been used to relieve pain, as well as for its antimicrobial and anti-inflammatory activity. Carnosol has assisted in the prevention of cartilage destruction, acted as a potent antioxidant and anti-inflammatory and reduced pro-inflammatory cytokines in studies too.

- **Resveratrol:** for those of you who swig a glass of red wine and offhandedly say it is 'for the good of your health', you are not wrong. There is a high concentration of resveratrol in grape skin and red wine, making it both anti-inflammatory and beneficial to immunity. Resveratrol has also shown joint-protective effects, controlling inflammation and protecting against RA and OA, and it may provide an alternative approach against the progression of inflammatory arthritis, such as RA.
- **Kaempferol:** kaempferol can be found in many edible plants, including the lovely leek and summer's sweet strawberry. It has the potential to be beneficial to the body in defending against inflammation and infection. It could be used in the future in the prevention and treatment of inflammatory diseases, such as RA, SLE, AS and even OA.
- **Soy (genistein):** the humble soybean, which contains genistein, has been found to have anti-inflammatory, pain-relieving and joint-protective properties, such as suppressing inflammation and reducing inflammatory cytokines. Used alongside methotrexate, genistein was found to be more effective than methotrexate alone in treating RA. Genistein-induced pain relief is being studied with its potential to attenuate the progression of OA.
- **Quercetin:** found in an array of foods, including onions tomatoes, cranberries and blackberries. My mum will be

pleased to know that it's even in capers. Organic tomatoes have been shown to have up to 79 per cent more quercetin than conventionally grown ones – a great incentive to begin growing a tomato plant at home. Effective against chronic diseases, including arthritis, quercetin is able to modulate and inhibit both acute and chronic inflammation.

Vital Vitamins and Marvellous Minerals

'Magnesium for sleep' or 'vitamin C for colds' . . . Is there any truth in this? Being deficient in vitamins and minerals can lead to a number of diseases in humans. As there are around 13 vitamins and 15 or so minerals, I will focus here on those that have the most relevance to arthritis, musculoskeletal disorders and autoimmunity.

Vitamin D

Vitamin D supports our immune system, has anti-inflammatory effects, strengthens our bones and is responsible for increasing the absorption of minerals. But across the world, around 1 billion people – of all ethnicities and ages – have been found to have low vitamin D levels. Vitamin D deficiency seems to be prevalent in RA, and at one time, my vitamin D levels were incredibly low. Low vitamin D intake appears also to be associated with an increased risk for OA progression.

We can retrieve small amounts of vitamin D naturally from our food (oily fish, egg yolks) or from the sun – so grab your sunhat, because sitting in the sun not only feels good, it does you good too.

Studies in Tenerife (what a lovely project for researchers!) suggested that wearing sunscreen does not hinder our vitamin D levels either, *so there is no excuse*. And the WHO recommends that casual sun exposure from 5 to 15 minutes, up to three times a week is sufficient (the darker your skin, the more sunlight you need, due to higher melanin levels that slow the production of vitamin D).

Vitamin C

When we think of vitamin C, we may picture citrus fruits, but numerous other fresh fruits and vegetables contain it, and native Australian superfood the Kakadu plum contains 100 times more vitamin C than oranges. Vitamin C has been shown to protect cartilage, prevent OA joint damage and lower levels of inflammation. It may protect against gout flare-ups too, and has properties similar to opioids, so could be used in the future for pain relief. Notably, people with the lowest intake of fruits and vegetables (less than 56mg of vitamin C – the equivalent of an orange or half a banana) have been associated with triple the risk of developing inflammatory arthritis too. When I think back to how little I cared for my body when my inflammatory arthritis took hold, this is unsurprising, even more so considering vitamin C's capacity for strengthening the immune system by fighting off colds and infectious diseases. (I was full of cold when my arthritis began!)

Selenium

Low selenium levels have been linked to an increased risk of RA and OA. How selenium may help RA or OA is not well understood, but it might be related to its antioxidant and anti-inflammatory properties, supporting our immunity. Selenium levels in foods are greatly dependent on the selenium content of the soil in which plants are grown, but Brazil nuts have the highest of all (see my dad's favourite snack, p. 152).

Zinc

Zinc is the second-most common mineral found in our bodies after iron. Vital to regulating the immune system, it exhibits antioxidant and anti-inflammatory activity. RA and AID patients appear to have significantly lower zinc levels compared to other people. Therapeutically, zinc reduces the duration and severity of common-cold symptoms too. So, it's worth getting some into your diet, for sure (it can be found in oysters, as well as other shellfish, meat, legumes such as chickpeas, nuts and seeds, and wholegrains such as oats). I definitely consume more of it in the winter months.

Magnesium

Magnesium can be found in our bones, and every cell, every organ and the immune system require it in order to function properly. It can readily be found in food (in raw cacao, avocados, nuts, seeds, legumes and leafy greens), as a supplement or a topical cream, but processed foods have a much lower content than unrefined products. Magnesium supplements have been linked to a number of benefits, including fighting inflammation, improving sleep and reducing stress. I adore an Epsom-salt bath, packed with magnesium (see pp. 173–5). Anecdotally, magnesium is said to provide pain relief from arthritic conditions. A topical methotrexate gel enriched with magnesium oil has even been shown to improve arthritic joint mobility, repair and decrease inflammation.

Good Fats

Fats (or fatty acids) store energy, insulate us and safeguard our vital organs. And, they start chemical reactions contributing to growth, immune function, reproduction and more. If this was not enough to keep fats busy, they also assist the body in stashing away certain nutrients, such as 'fat-soluble' vitamins A, D, E and K. Central to how all humans regulate their energy is the making, breaking, storing and deploying of fats, and an imbalance in this can result in disease.

Fats are usually saturated or unsaturated – or a combination of both. A small amount of fat is an essential part of a healthy, balanced diet, but for long-term health, some fats are better than others. High-quality 'good' fats included in this chapter are monounsaturated and polyunsaturated. Inflammatory ones include industrial-made trans fats, while saturated fats fall somewhere in the middle, and can be found in the next chapter.

Unsaturated fats

Good fats (monounsaturated or polyunsaturated) are derived in the main from vegetables, nuts, seeds and fatty fish. These fats are liquid at room temperature, rather than solid like saturated fats. Replacing saturated fats with unsaturated fats has substantial health benefits.

Monounsaturated fats

The Mediterranean diet is rich in antioxidants, with very low levels of saturated fats and high levels of mono- and polyunsaturated fats. High-monounsaturated diets can reduce inflammation, significantly lower inflammatory markers and suppress disease activity in RA patients. A high intake of saturated fat may be associated with increased progression of OA too, while high intake of mono- and polyunsaturated fats may be linked to reduced progression. The MD is regarded as the healthiest way to eat today, whether you have arthritis or not. Show me the olive oil!

Polyunsaturated fats

The two main types of polyunsaturated fatty acids are omega-3 and 6. Western diets are deficient in omega-3 and have excessive amounts of omega-6. It would be oversimplifying to consider omega-3 'good' and omega-6 'bad', as the body requires both. But a higher concentration of omega-6 in our systems could be pro-inflammatory, whereas higher levels of omega-3 may be anti-inflammatory. Some researchers propose that the omega-6/omega-3 ratio may have considerable implications for the development of many chronic diseases, including inflammatory ones and AIDs, but the optimal ratio has not been well assessed or established. For now, the advice would be to focus on omega-3s, especially as preliminary studies have shown promising effects for inflammatory and arthritic conditions like RA and OA. The three most important types are ALA, DHA and EPA:

- **ALA** The most common omega-3 fatty acid and the most essential, this is mainly found in plant foods and certain nuts. Chia seeds are a superb source, with around 65 per cent of the oil they contain being attributed to ALA.
- **DHA and EPA** These are produced via ALA or consumed directly from foods and/or dietary supplements (think omega-3 fish-oil capsules). Fish oil or fatty fish are substantial sources.

Good Gut Additions – Probiotics

The world of probiotics is fast becoming as diverse as the bacteria it encompasses. It's getting increasingly difficult to determine where to buy them and how to take them and harder to understand whether or not they will help us with our symptoms.

What are probiotics?

Described by WHO as 'live microorganisms that, when administered in adequate amounts, confer a health benefit on the host', probiotics consist mainly of bacteria or yeasts, are naturally present in fermented foods, may be added to other foods and are also available as dietary supplements.

What do they do?

Encouraging 'good' bacteria, they improve the natural balance of bacteria and function of our guts, and restore this balance when it has been disrupted by illness or through medicinal treatment.

How do they work?

Anecdotally, probiotics have numerous benefits, but in order for them to work, you need to keep eating them, as mostly they are transient (passing through the gut) rather than resident (staying put in the gut). Probiotics are not assured to provide the same effects for everyone, so if you are looking to introduce a supplement, speak to a health professional first, and pick up more fermented foods (yoghurt, kefir, sauerkraut, tempeh, miso, sourdough, to name a few) in the meantime.

Could they help inflammatory conditions?

Probiotics are a possible therapy for the treatment of inflammation-based arthritic conditions and AIDs, but there are only a few high-quality studies on the efficacy of fermented foods and probiotics in humans in general. Over time, scientists will unravel the complex interrelationships between the gut, immunity and arthritis, but further studies are required.

Fundamental Fibre

The foundation of plant-based wholefoods, from legumes to vegetables, fruits, wholegrains, nuts and seeds is fibre and they all contain more than 100 types of it. The recommendation of 30g fibre per day equates to at least two pieces of fruit, five portions of vegetables, three portions of wholegrains or one to two portions of nuts, seeds and legumes. And we should be consuming at least 30 different fibre-rich plant foods per week (although any increase in fibre should be undertaken gradually, making sure you are drinking enough water too – at least 3–4 litres per day). A high-fibre diet helps to promote a healthier gut, which is fundamental to the immune system, lower levels of inflammation and good mental and physical health.

Add These to Your Day: A Quick-reference Guide
Epigallocatechin gallate
Matcha powder, green tea
Curcumin
Turmeric root, turmeric powder
Gingerol
Ground ginger, fresh ginger, dried ginger
Hydroxytyrosol
Extra virgin olive oil, olives
Cinnamaldehyde
Cinnamon sticks, ground cinnamon powder
Carnosol
Rosemary, sage, thyme, marjoram, basil, oregano
Resveratrol
Peanuts, cranberries, pistachios, blueberries, bilberries, grapes, grape juice, red wine, cacao powder
Kaempferol
Tea, broccoli, cabbage, kale, beans, endives, tomatoes, grapes, botanical products traditionally used in medicine such as *Moringa oleifera*

Genistein
Soy-containing foods: tofu, soya milk, soya flour, soy protein, tempeh, miso; legumes like chickpeas (small amounts)
Quercetin
Onions, capers, apples, grapes, berries, broccoli, citrus fruits, cherries, green tea, capers, cacao, lingonberries, bilberries, blackcurrants
Vitamin D
UV rays from the sun, egg yolks, fatty fish like salmon or tuna, supplements (cod-liver oil)
Vitamin C
Acerola cherries, chilli peppers, guavas, blackcurrants, thyme, kale, kiwis, broccoli, strawberries, citrus fruits, Kakadu plum
Selenium
Brazil nuts, fish, meat and eggs
Zinc
Nuts – Brazil, pine, cashews, pecans; seeds – squash, pumpkin, sunflower, chia, flax; meat; shellfish (oysters); legumes (chickpeas); wholegrains (oats)
Magnesium
Water, leafy green vegetables, fruits, nuts (almonds, cashews, Brazil nuts), seeds (flax, chia, pumpkin) and unprocessed wholegrains (wheat, oats, quinoa), legumes (lentils, beans, chickpeas), fish and meat
Monounsaturated fatty acids
Olive oil, olives, avocados, sesame seeds, almonds, cashews, hazelnuts, peanuts, pistachios (plus oils or spreads made from)

Polyunsaturated fatty acids: omega-3 (ALA)
Chia seeds, vegetable oils, linseed (flaxseed), nuts (walnuts, pecans and hazelnuts) and green leafy vegetables
Polyunsaturated fatty acids: omega-3 (EPA and DHA)
Fish oil or fatty fish such as salmon, mackerel, anchovies
Probiotics
Yoghurt, kefir, sauerkraut, tempeh, kimchi, miso, kombucha, cottage cheese, pickles, sourdough
You will find the majority of the above in the recipes in Chapter 5 (see p. 85).

3

Avoiding Inflammation

'All disease begins in the gut.'
Hippocrates of Kos, physician

The antitheses of inflammation-fighting foods are inflammation-inducing foods, and goodness knows, I can tell when I have had one too many.

It's worth trying to move away from thoughts of 'good' and 'bad' food, and instead to consider 'better' food and better choices we can make for our bodies. There is no instant fix, but there are ways to do some fixing. Consider this chapter (and the book as a whole) as an educational toolbox. It is handing you the tools to make alternative choices for your health, rather than restricting your choices. It's about lifestyle *adjustments*. It is not as basic as 'I can never eat a deep-fried doughnut again' (I know how tasty they can be), just that there is *probably* a more nourishing alternative – and there are *loads* of alternatives. Your gut microbiota, mind and body will thank you for making better choices.

What Is Inflammation, Anyway?

We've talked a lot so far about inflammation, but not about what it actually is. Given the bad press it gets, you might be surprised to learn that inflammation in a normally functioning immune system is actually a positive thing. It is the process by which your immune system both recognises and defends against unwanted visitors (like infections) and repairs damage. Usually short lived and found at the site of injury or infection – whether a scarlet stubbed toe or a scratchy sore throat – this is known as acute inflammation. It is a clever, unconscious function, which acts when required and slumbers when it is not.

If inflammation switches to sleep-walking mode, however, continuing to operate beneath the surface, it is no longer working as it is supposed to. Inflammation like this is low-grade and chronic. Signs and symptoms are less obvious than the normal inflammation we see in our bodies. Chronic inflammation manifests in the form of pain (typically in the joints), anxiety and depression (inflammation affects the whole body, including the brain) and fatigue (connected to stress). When inflammation persists for a long time it can lead to many chronic diseases, including cancer, cardiovascular, neurodegenerative or respiratory diseases – and, you guessed it, arthritis.

Arthritis, as we have established, is associated with excess levels of inflammation in the body. If we imagine this as an ongoing fire within us, low-grade or not, it will be wreaking havoc. And throwing in an abundance of inflammatory foods, a sprinkling of stress, a week's worth of inadequate sleep and no exercise could be compared to pouring fuel all over this inner fire, causing it to burn even more ferociously.

Becoming a fire tamer

If we just focus on diet for now, simply adding one anti-inflammatory food to your daily intake – like that shot of juice I mentioned in Chapter 2 – would not be enough to tame the fire. Especially when you are simultaneously still splashing on the fuel, whether in the form of junk food, alcohol or sleepless nights.

The objective here, then, is to eliminate the fuel completely (it may take time, and it may not be all the time, but it is possible) and replace it with a fire-engine-style hose-down – not in the form of 100 shots of turmeric or ginger, no, but by consuming an array of colourful plant-based wholefoods (along with modifications to lifestyle, treatment plans, sleep and more).

The inflammation may not disappear completely – after all, we are talking about a chronic inflammatory immune response here, so it is more complicated than this – but perhaps your inner inflammation might become calmer and more manageable than it was and, as a consequence, you could end up finding some relief from your symptoms. You've got this – you're a fire tamer now!

Food and Inflammation

It is uncertain exactly *how* certain foods and substances affect the human body in relation to arthritis, AIDs and inflammatory conditions, but the research is developing (in the form of the expansion of psychobiotic research – see Chapter 9). That is why it is worth recalling my previous nod to us all being individual human beings who all react differently, based on (put simply) genetics, gut microbiome, lifestyle and immunity. The aim, then, is to use this chapter to address things that may exacerbate *your* condition in *your* body.

The standard American diet (SAD) and the Western pattern diet (WPD) are largely weight-gaining and highly inflammatory, characterised by a high content of meat, ultra-processed foods, saturated fats, refined produce, sugar, alcohol and an associated reduced consumption of fruits and vegetables, with barely any fibre. A lot of (but not all) inflammatory foods are weight-gaining (no surprise there), and substantial evidence has surfaced making it clear that obesity is associated with chronic low-level inflammation. So, the more excess weight you have, the more inflamed you are likely to be.

A worldwide obesity epidemic is the direct result of on-demand, highly accessible and mass-produced products, or 'junk food': cheap, sugar-filled beverages and ultra-processed or refined foods that are high in salt, sugar, additives (E-numbers), saturated or trans fats. Think processed meats or cheeses (cheese single slices, bacon, sausages, salami), refined grains (white bread, cakes, biscuits), pre-made produce (microwave or ready meals, grab-and-go sandwiches), processed beverages (sweetened juices, pasteurised cow's milk, milkshakes), confectionery (sweets, chocolate bars), ice cream, jam and salty snacks (crisps, sausage rolls, pies and pasties). These food types provide only a short-term feeling of fullness with potentially damaging long-term effects.

What exactly is the damage?

In order to explore the damaging effects of junk food on the gut, professor of genetic epidemiology Tim Spector convinced his son Tom to embark on a fast-food/junk-fest diet for ten days. Unsurprisingly, Tom did not feel well on it – and neither did his gut microbes, which had taken on an inflammatory function. The diversity of his gut microbiome plummeted and looked how any junk-food eater's might.

Inflammation and illness-causing chemicals have been demonstrated to increase by about 70 per cent with a high-fat, low-fibre diet; but the good news is that switching to a Mediterranean-style anti-inflammatory diet for 30 days does reverse the damage. High-fat, high-sugar diets are shown to increase inflammation, and can affect brain health (for more about the gut–brain connection, see p. 238). Obesity, alcohol, tobacco and poor diet have all been associated with an increased risk of inflammatory rheumatic conditions, and inflammation-induced chronic diseases. Eating in a more anti-inflammatory way is not only beneficial for your arthritis, but for your body overall.

Face the fats

Like inflammation, fats have a bad reputation, as demonstrated by the plethora of fat-free yoghurts, low-fat foods and 'light' versions of the full-fat original foods. But fats, as we saw in Chapter 2 (see pp. 40–42), are vital for a range of functions, the specific purpose depending upon their type. To recap, most foods incorporate a mix of saturated and unsaturated fats, with some being higher in one than the other.

Saturated fatty acids

A reasonable and modest intake of saturated fat should not be an alarming health concern – anything in moderation is not typically harmful – but, if you start eating like Tom Spector (see p. 50), it will alter your microbiota and your health.

Saturated fats (fats that are solid at room temperature) are mainly found in animal sources including red meat, poultry and full-fat dairy products (whole milk, butter and cream). They may also be found in coconut oil (which is less likely to promote inflammation) – and palm oil (found in almost 50 per cent of the packaged products found in grocery stores, from cereals, pizza, doughnuts and chocolate to deodorant, shampoo, toothpaste and lipstick).

Regular and heavy consumption of foods containing saturated fats does cause harm to our health, triggering a damaging inflammatory response (we do not need that) and gut distress. Notably though, not all saturated fats are the same and those in certain types of dairy – namely cheese and yoghurt – may not be as harmful as others. A focus on more unsaturated fats than saturated, and on the good kind of saturated fats, underpins the healthful, anti-inflammatory MD.

Trans fatty acids

Broadly speaking, there are two types of trans fats found in foods: naturally occurring and artificial. Naturally, they are found in small amounts in certain animal products. Artificial trans fats are industrially produced oils that may be used to provide a longer shelf life for food, or as a cooking oil to deep-fry fast foods. Artificial trans fats have been identified as one of the most dangerous food additives, associated with excess levels of inflammation and more. In fact, the WHO is occupied with eliminating them from the global food supply by 2023.

Refined and processed foods

The word 'refined' suggests sophistication and elegance, and a secondary definition is to purify a substance into a finer form – like refining gold. But the way I see it, refined foods may be refined in the sense that they have been stripped and purified, but this is a process that rids them of their best qualities – their original (and natural) nutrient content, including vitamins, minerals and fibre. Highly processed refined ingredients are easy to identify, with their chalk white and colourless appearance: white flour, white sugar, etc. And they form the basis of many processed foods such as white breads, pizza dough, pasta, pastries, cakes and cookies. There is even refined sugar lurking in your 'healthy' cereal.

White rice is not bad, and it is cheaper to buy and quicker to cook too. But wholegrain brown rice, red rice, black rice or wild rice would triumph hands down in a nutritional contest, with numerous nutrients and lower GIs. The glycaemic index, or GI, is used to measure the increase in blood glucose (sugar) levels from the foods we eat: any carbohydrate-rich foods we eat show up in our bloodstream as glucose, the body's prime source of energy. Some carbohydrates are digested and absorbed into the bloodstream quickly (high-GI) and others more slowly (low-GI).

High-GI foods such as processed foods, as well as white potatoes and sugary soft drinks, are rapidly digested and cause considerable fluctuations in blood-glucose and insulin levels. A diet based on high-GI foods has been shown to cause and worsen inflammation, whereas low-GI foods like wholegrain breads, brown rice, legumes, quinoa and sweet potatoes take longer to digest, producing gradual rises in blood glucose and insulin levels. A Mediterranean-style, low-GI diet is ideal for controlling inflammation. Nutritional therapist Victoria Jain adds that avoiding added sugars and refined carbohydrates is key to managing symptoms of arthritis.

A spoonful of sugar

Processing for foods ranges from the traditional methods (heat treatment, fermentation, pickling, drying, curing, smoking) to more modern ones (pasteurisation, ultra-heat treatment, high-pressure processing or modified-atmosphere packaging) and is usually for the purpose of extending shelf life. But it is also to make the food taste more palatable. And sugar is the staple.

It is nigh-on impossible to find packaged products in the supermarket that *don't* have added sugar or sweeteners. We crave sugar. It gives us a buzz. It tastes good. We want more. But then we look up and realise we have finished the whole slab of chocolate that we'd planned on putting back into the fridge to save for tomorrow.

Sugar has addictive properties and long-term overuse of it in our diets can have devastating consequences on health over time, including the potential to make us inflamed and depressed too – two issues many of us are already contending with daily.

By now, you have probably realised that reducing your refined-sugar intake or ditching it for good is as beneficial for your health as it is for your wellbeing. But sugar is sugar – whether white, refined or unrefined 'natural' sugar, they all have a similar reaction in the body. However, certain types of unrefined sugar might actually be good for you, and best of all, bees, plants and trees do the work for us, making sweet syrups: honey, agave, date, molasses and maple.

Honey is marvellous and humans have had a fondness for honey bees and their produce as far back as the Stone Age. Containing trace amounts of several vitamins and minerals, high-quality honey exudes antioxidant and anti-inflammatory phytonutrients and prebiotic activity. However, these health benefits are specific to raw, real and unpasteurised honey; the honey found in grocery stores is usually pasteurised. So, go local rather than mass-produced whenever possible.

A note on salt

Salt is vital to us, but just as there is excessive consumption of sugar, salt – naturally found in meat and regularly added to preserved foods – is following closely behind. Worldwide, the average consumption of salt per day is 9–12g, but the recommended requirement is a mere 3.75g (or two-thirds of a teaspoon). Too much salt intake is associated with a higher risk of developing RA and numerous studies have established that it induces and aggravates AIDs.

Reading by E-numbers: food additives

Emulsifiers, preservatives, artificial sweeteners, stabilisers, thickeners, bulking agents or extracted colours and antioxidants are all food additives labelled with a number with an 'E' prefix. The list of E-numbers is exactly 338 numbers long, and they all exist in our packaged foods. Some are extracted from natural sources, but many are chemically derived, and at the time of writing, there is still so much we don't know about these or the real effects that they have on our guts – and thus our immune systems (see 'Proceed with Caution', below).

Emulsifiers make it possible for water and oil to blend together to produce a stable and smooth emulsion. Some are found naturally, in eggs, nuts and soybeans, but industrial food processors may use commercial ones that harm the mucus lining and microbe content of your gut, inducing low-grade inflammation, among other things. We don't need any more inflammation, do we?

Artificial Sweeteners

As sugar has been proven to increase the risk of a number of diseases, how do manufacturers navigate this in an inexpensive way, while replicating the taste and feeling that the real deal provides? By producing artificial alternatives, of course. Acesulfame K, aspartame, saccharin, sorbitol, sucralose (Splenda), stevia and xylitol – ranging from about 180 times sweeter to as much as 13,000 times sweeter than sugar – are all low-calorie or calorie-free chemical substances used to sweeten a plethora of products, from drinks to desserts, and even toothpaste.

The ingestion of artificial sweeteners has been shown to alter our guts, with an almost 50 per cent decrease in the number and diversity of beneficial gut bacteria. As we are aware already, optimal gut health is paramount to maintaining a healthy immune system and bodily functions. Artificial sweeteners promote 'bad' bacteria and inflammation, with similar effects shown for sucralose, and we arthritics do not need any more inflammation in our bodies. Although some of these findings are from studies conducted on animals, all these additives potentially have implications for humans with inflammatory diseases.

PROCEED WITH CAUTION

Most of the chemical safety testing of food additives and sweeteners focuses on determining the toxicity (risk of death, poisoning or cancer), not on changes in our bodies, or on the gut. Until we understand more about the inner effects of food additives, it might be wise to reduce or avoid these seemingly 'harmless' chemicals. Moreover, for those of us living with AIDs, Victoria Jain writes that eating foods that contain toxins or foreign substances, such as synthetic sweeteners and other additives (as mentioned above), can cause the body to become overwhelmed, leading to inflammation as they overstimulate the immune system, switching it to hyperdrive.

Try Plant Milks

In 2018, scientists in Florida discovered that a strain of bacteria found in milk and beef could be a trigger for developing RA in those genetically at risk. More research is needed, but it does make me wonder about the meat that was one of the triggers leading to my condition and if I am genetically predisposed.

Fortunately, there are endless types of plant milks now, from almond to tigernut and more (see p. 85). You can even make almond milk yourself at home: just blend and strain almonds soaked in water.

Glorifying Gluten-Free: Should We?

Gluten-free products are popping up all over the shop, from breads and cakes to all sorts of snacks. Gluten-free is being glorified. But we need to look at what gluten is being replaced with. And whether we are in danger of following a hyped trend in order to avoid it?

Gluten is a dietary protein found in grains such as wheat, barley and rye or in products containing them. It's what makes bread and pizza doughs so sticky and malleable. Processed and high-GI products form a large part of our diets. Wheat-based cereal for breakfast with a teaspoon of sugar, followed by a grab-and-go 'healthy' sandwich for lunch and a pasta bake for dinner used to be a typical daily diet for me. But choosing gluten-free versions of typical old-me foods would not be conducive to helping gut microbiome diversity; in fact, it would probably make it worse. Going gluten-free is not about replicating gluten-containing foods, but rather replacing them – substituting that hefty processed white bread with nourishing vegetables, for example. Recipes in this book are largely gluten-free or have gluten-free options to cater for all, so you can track and see if the removal of gluten has any an impact on your overall health or symptoms.

You may have heard of the 'leaky gut', a normal bodily function whereby the gut becomes more 'leaky', allowing the body to absorb what it needs from the digestive tract. But this intestinal permeability can lead to microscopic damage linked to a number of diseases, including RA. My advice is to trial and test to see what works for you, keep a food diary (see pp. 82–4) and speak to a doctor or nutritionist if you are concerned.

Alcohol: Going it Sober Isn't So Bad

Alcohol is embedded into many cultures, and if you tell someone you do not drink or are not going to drink, they'll sometimes look at you like you're an extraterrestrial being from another planet: shocked, because even though things appear to be changing, most people do drink alcohol; fascinated, at your confidence in countering public opinion; slightly terrified, at the realisation that you will remember the evening, whereas they probably will not . . . But it's not always like this, and the way people react often says more about them than it does about you. In my experience, most people are comfortable with it, supportive even, ordering me a 'mocktail' and possibly even joining me in not drinking.

If anyone tries to pressure you into drinking, makes you feel uncomfortable or as though you have done something wrong, stand your ground and remember: it is their insecurities and their problem if they are unable to respect your boundaries. Your choices for your body, mind and wellbeing deserve respect. Always.

Having been prescribed methotrexate, I had to significantly reduce my weekly alcohol consumption from the age of 22 (my rheumatologist initially advised none at all). I found it hard when it seemed drinking was all my friends did for fun at the time. As you mature, however, hangovers are less appealing and take longer to recover from. I never 'miss out' on the fun of socialising by not drinking, but I do (gladly) miss out on wasting weekends hungover, meaning that, unlike some of my friends, I wake up fresh as a daisy (if a little tired). You can still join your friends in bars, have an occasional glass of red wine, or something else when you feel like it. I know I do sometimes, all the while knowing that these external choices are having an internal effect on my health. Swapping a hard spirit served with a carbonated, sugar-filled fizzy mixer for a wholesome glass of organic red wine with its rich anti-inflammatory polyphenolic content may make all the difference. Heavy or binge quantities of alcohol can increase inflammation in the body though, and even small amounts have effects on sleep quality (see p. 222) and immunity. Overconsumption may increase the risk of certain types of arthritis too (if you don't already have it).

You may have discovered that alcohol aggravates your symptoms. Any time I consumed or overconsumed alcohol in the past, I would feel it the following day. Many medicines prescribed to relieve arthritis symptoms do not combine well with alcohol, including NSAIDs (see p. 20), which carry a greater risk for stomach bleeding and ulcers when you drink. DMARDs (like methotrexate), biologics and alcohol can make you more susceptible to liver damage.

Smoking or Non-Smoking?

I remember walking into restaurants, pubs and bars as a child, and my parents being asked, 'Smoking or Non-Smoking?' Nowadays, the thought of someone puffing away while you are trying to eat is a bit absurd!

Smoking (yourself or passively) increases the risk of developing more than 50 serious health conditions, and promotes certain AIDs like RA or PsA. It has damaging effects on our bones and joints, impactful no matter the type of arthritis that you have. Unsurprisingly, it impairs our defences and promotes autoimmunity, with heavy smokers, who smoked 20 a day for at least 20 years, having a more than two-and-a-half times increased risk of the most severe form of RA. But the good news is that after 15 years of quitting for good, the risk decreases by a third.

But what about if you already have arthritis or RA? Smoking can exacerbate your symptoms and interfere with the effectiveness of your medications or treatments. If you require surgery, smoking may increase the chances of complications and impact your recovery post-surgery. You may also not be aware that your smoking is making your symptoms worse even if it provides you with a temporary calm. So, if you are a smoker and you want to improve your symptoms – or decrease your chance of other health problems – it's time to stub out the cig once and for all. Speak to your GP about quitting, and they will be able to equip you with the right support to help you do it.

Anecdotal Antidotes for Arthritis

Starting on the Arthritis Foodie journey felt like standing at the entrance to a humongous overgrown maze with multiple pathways, in the dark and without a map. There was no indication as to which path led where and if I would be taken down the right track or not: don't eat nightshade plants (what is a nightshade plant, anyway?); don't eat dairy (but a probiotic like kefir might be all right, just avoid lactose); cut out gluten, eggs and refined sugar; remove everything processed; stop eating acidic foods (like citrus fruits – but you *can* have apple cider vinegar, lots of that); go vegan; go carnivorous – wait, no, actually, don't eat red meat (or maybe you can occasionally, if its grass-fed and organic); watch your pH balance – choose alkaline foods; you should really stop eating peanut butter – in fact, all nuts and seeds; deep-fried food? Absolutely not; and 'gluten ain't great', but additives and preservatives are *far worse* . . .

Some of this was relevant and a lot of it was simply not supported by science (at least not yet). I did try *all* of it though. Every arthritis-anti-inflammatory-autoimmune protocol, book and idea for improving chronic arthritis and inflammatory conditions – I collected them all, absorbed them and tested them. All of which means that, as I have done the bulk of the legwork for you, this book is a much simpler guide and support for you as you move forward on your journey.

What we can be sure of is that there is currently *no* scientific evidence to support the following: avoiding nightshades (such as tomatoes, peppers and aubergines), overconsuming apple cider vinegar, cutting out nuts and seeds, eggs or citrus fruits, being carnivorous, eating 'alkaline'-only foods – and the list goes on (as you've seen). If trying and testing any of these helps you, then go for it, but as noted already, the MD appears to be the most science-supported diet known to us: naturally anti-inflammatory, it has the most potential to battle with us against the chronic inflammatory and autoimmune diseases so prevalent in the world today. One study in particular concluded that the MD diet reduced inflammation in RA patients with an improvement in vitality and physical functions. Unhealthy lifestyles and detrimental diets contribute unquestionably to the rise of inflammatory diseases and autoimmunity in the populations of both developed and developing countries. Diet is intrinsically attached to socioeconomic status, and often the healthier options are more expensive and less accessible or too time-consuming, which is a disheartening problem (and one too big for me to tackle in this book, but it's important to mention).

As we've seen, there is no one-size-fits-all approach, but what I have provided you with is everything that has helped me and been proven to help in early-stage or advanced studies in relation to arthritis. There *are* multiple pathways to relieving inflammation, but unlike my maze, yours is now trimmed, the sun is out and all the paths are leading to the same destination. You are at the start of your maze and, with this guide in your hand, all you have to do is place one foot in front of the other. And enjoy the *delicious* food that comes with that.

Easy Swaps: A Quick-Reference Guide
If it is feeling overwhelming, here are some quick wins for your dinner plate – what to cut back on and how to replace it.
✗Refined white, processed breads and buns
✓Sourdough bread, seed-based bread, oat cakes, brown rice cakes
✗Refined and processed breakfast cereals
✓Porridge, plus go-to 'Breakfast' (see pp. 90–101)
✗White rice and white potatoes
✓Nutrient-dense brown, red, black and wild rice, quinoa, beans and legumes and sweet potatoes
✗Commercially processed baked goods: doughnuts, biscuits, cakes, cookies and chocolate bars
✓Bake your own delicious treats (see 'Desserts, snacks and treats', pp.141–152)
✗Refined sugar, and sugary sweets
✓Honey, maple, date, agave syrups; or make your own snacks

✗Deep-fried foods and trans-fat fried crisps (or chips)
✓Wholefoods are really the only replacement for junk food. For savoury replacements try olives, crispy kale (see p. 105) or hummus (see p. 165); and try sliced apple with peanut butter, or flavoured nuts (see p. 141)
✗Pizza
✓If you are craving pizza, try a tomato-based sourdough pizza with loads of vegetables; otherwise, use an omelette as your 'pizza' base and top accordingly
✗Pasta
✓Reduce your intake of refined flour by replacing it with brown rice-noodle dishes or using brown rice/quinoa/spelt/buckwheat flour pasta
✗Pre-prepared meals, such as soups or sandwiches
✓Be wary of the additives – only some brands are fresh and transparent about ingredients; otherwise try soup recipes (see pp. 102–4)
✗Dairy products
✓See how you feel, but as mentioned, dairy such as kefir or natural yoghurt (due to the breakdown in lactose) has anti- rather than pro-inflammatory effects
✗Alcohol
✓Red organic wine, alcohol-free lookalikes or abstention – just be wary of sugar intake and balance with H20
✗Fizzy drinks
✓Add fresh fruit and herbs to a cold bottle of mineral water for a delicious refresher or use fruity tea leaves to make iced tea

4

Putting A Plan In Place

'A goal without a plan is just a wish.'
Antoine de Saint-Exupéry, writer, aviator'

Before Arthritis Foodie, I rarely prepared food 'from scratch' and I was not great at cooking. 'Arthritis diets', 'diets for arthritis', 'anti-inflammatory recipes', 'healthy food', 'plant-based recipes', books, bloggers and bestsellers . . . At first, I felt bewildered and I did not have much confidence in myself. How on earth I was going to do this? The recipes I found looked healthy and sounded delicious, but, *honestly* – I thought I'd have to be a Michelin-starred chef to produce any of them. I hardly recognised many of the ingredients listed, unsure what they looked like, let alone how to cook them. And my seasoning shelf consisted of salt, pepper, chilli flakes and one small container of 'Italian Mixed Herbs'. My kitchen was not equipped for cooking from scratch. And neither was I.

Recipe books often expect you to have and know it all, which is very complimentary of the authors – but not exactly realistic and perhaps a bit presumptuous. I made a list, writing down all the equipment I'd require and picking out threads of common ingredients I would need. That list detailed everything from spices to seeds, herbs to honey and tea to tempeh. I even wrote down 'chickpea water' – like it was an item I could buy. This was obviously before I learned that 'chickpea water' is simply the leftover liquid from a can of chickpeas *in* water. Oh dear, I had a lot to learn!

Back then, I could not grasp what 'wholefood recipes' really meant. But eventually, experimenting recipe by recipe, I discovered flavoursome foods, vibrant colours and a joy in cooking from scratch. The difference I feel in eating and living this way has been tremendous. Impactful enough to have led me to write this book for you, in the hope that you can feel its benefits too. This is not cooking for dummies, and I do not want to patronise anyone; but these sections have been written with someone in mind – past *me*. It includes all the details I wish someone had put into layman's terms for me when I started on the Arthritis Foodie journey, because I just did not know where to begin and *I know* how you might be feeling now. Here is the beginning I wish I had had.

Everything You Need

Cooking equipment

- **Y-shaped peeler** A hand-held, Y-shaped, wide, sturdy and strong peeler is easier to use when your hands are hurting or swollen.

- **Avocado slicer** I had an avocado-hand mishap (I cut my hand open removing a stone from an avocado, as I am heavy handed and clumsy) and I do not want this happening to any of you. My hand was out of action for almost a month. Please use this slicer/stone remover/scooper tool!
- **Blender** You will use this all time. The one made by Breville is not too expensive, lasts for years and does not take up too much room. You will be making five-minute breakfast smoothies, iced matcha lattes and cashew-nut pasta sauces in no time.
- **Large cooking pot** Essentially, a non-stick shallow casserole dish (26 or 30cm in diameter). Make sure that it can be also used on a hob, because some are made for oven use only.
- **Oven Pyrex dish** For those extra-crispy roasted vegetables or baked chocolate brownies. An essential for the kitchen.
- **Non-stick trays** An assortment of sizes and depths is recommended for any oven-based cooking or baking.
- **Measuring jug** A strong Pyrex one, with all the different units you need from litres to pints.
- **Weighing scales** Any will do, but I prefer the battery-powered type because they provide a more precise measurement reading.
- **Food processor** The processor I have at home has three different set-ups: a small blender that works like a pestle and mortar, a medium-sized blender and a large food processer. The food processer has grating and peeling settings too.

GO-TO GADGETS

The world does not always consider the arthritic hand, or wrist, or arm, but luckily, some creative designers have. So, why not let gadgets do the work for you, so that you don't have to – or at least only with minimal effort and reduced pain. Here are some of the inventions that might help you in the kitchen:

- Angled large grip knives
- Electric tin opener
- Silicone grips for opening jars and bottles
- One-cup kettle
- Compression gloves
- Automatic electric stirrers

Utensils

Aside from the standard cutlery and wooden spoons, there are some tools that will make your life easier when it comes to cooking.

- Spatulas, stirring spoons, serving spoons and a potato masher
- Flat silicone spatula
- Kitchen tongs
- Hand-held electric whisk

Additional essentials

- Glass mixing bowls – a range of three sizes
- Range of pans: griddle pan, frying pans and a wok
- Sieve and colander
- Food-storage containers

Essential Foods

From week to week, recipe to recipe, the foods you are cooking with will change, but these are the staple items that I like to have in my fridge, freezer and store cupboard, because usually something flavoursome can be easily rustled up with them.

When you are in pain, having a flare-up or simply not in the mood to think about cooking, having these items at the ready will help. Many a time you'll find me sitting at the kitchen table, my ankles wrapped up in heat packs, chopping vegetables and throwing them together in a pan with a spice mix. Or getting a helping hand from my friends and family.

Fresh/frozen

- Plant milk
- Red onions
- Bananas
- Apples
- Eggs
- Avocados
- Sweet potatoes
- Courgettes
- Salmon
- Carrots
- Broccoli
- Kale
- Frozen spinach
- Frozen peas
- Frozen raspberries
- Frozen blueberries
- Frozen bulk-made recipes (such as mushroom soup or chickpea curry)

Store-cupboard essentials

If this next list is too much for you to purchase in one go, just buy items as and when you see them in a recipe. For me, it is a relief to know that I can cook absolutely anything from home by just getting in fresh ingredients from week to week and topping up the dry store-cupboard – e.g. more quinoa or tins of chickpeas.

With all of the below, I choose 100 per cent wholefoods wherever possible – no processing, additives or added salt and sugar. If I am able to buy organic and can afford to, then I do that too.

Oils, vinegars and sauces

- Extra virgin olive oil
- Coconut oil
- Sesame oil
- Balsamic vinegar
- Apple cider vinegar
- Molasses
- Tamari (or soy sauce, if not accessible)
- Tomato purée

Beans, pulses and other tins

- Cannellini beans in water
- Chickpeas in water
- Tinned coconut milk
- Butter beans in water
- Red kidney beans in water
- Chopped tomatoes

Dry goods

- Porridge oats (note: if highly sensitive to gluten, choose oats that have not been packaged in a gluten-producing setting)
- Quinoa
- Gluten-free pasta (red lentil, brown rice)
- Brown rice
- Red split lentils

- Rice noodles
- Gluten-free flour options: brown rice, buckwheat, oat, coconut
- Kallo stock cubes
- Nutritional yeast
- Polenta
- Baking powder

Herbs, spices and powders

- Garlic cloves
- Root ginger (keep a piece in the freezer and chop from there)
- Moringa powder
- Ground turmeric
- Ground ginger
- Garlic granules
- Ground cumin
- Paprika
- Smoked paprika
- Garam masala
- Garlic granules
- Chilli powder/flakes
- Cayenne pepper
- Mild curry powder
- Cardamom pods/powder
- Ground coriander
- Rosemary
- Thyme
- Oregano
- Coriander leaf
- Star anise
- Chipotle chilli flakes
- Garam masala
- Dried harissa spices
- Cayenne chilli pepper
- Ground allspice
- Ground nutmeg
- Baking powder
- Cinnamon
- Dried mint
- Italian herbs blend
- Black pepper
- Sea salt

Oats, nuts and seeds

- Black or brown mustard seeds
- Whole cumin seeds
- Coriander seeds

- Porridge oats
- Chia seeds
- Ground flaxseeds
- Ground almonds
- Sesame seeds
- Cashew nuts (for sauces)
- Pine nuts (for pesto)
- Mixed nuts (i.e. bags of mixed nuts for snacks – containing walnuts, almonds, Brazil nuts, pecans, cashew nuts)

Sweet, savoury and teas

- Honey
- Manuka honey
- Maple syrup
- Peanut butter
- Desiccated coconut
- Coconut sugar
- Date syrup
- Peanut butter
- Raw cacao powder
- Dates
- Matcha powder
- Green tea

A guide to what's in your 65 recipes

Day zero of Arthritis Foodie. Crisp, colourful and clean cookbooks were amassed on my shelf – as new as the sense of responsibility I had acquired for my health. And what a responsibility! The thought that I really could make a difference to my wellbeing with all these recipes and remedies. Taking one from my shelf, I slowly turned the pages to choose some recipes for the week – kale and quinoa salad, a chia-seed-topped porridge, a curry using mustard seeds and served with wild rice . . . It might as well have been written in a foreign language for all that I understood or recognised. Honestly, what was kale? How were chia seeds used? What did 'superfood' mean? And, I had no idea how to pronounce quinoa, never mind how to cook with it.

Well, this chapter provides the answers to all those questions and more. Below, I have described ingredients that you may not yet have heard of, so you can get to know them ahead of the recipes that they appear in. For any unfamiliar spices or herbs, flip back to Chapter 2. Oh – and I use the word 'superfood' when referring to a particular food item that is relatively more dense in nutrients compared to others (and there are plenty of them in this book). Please note that the superfoods have been marked with: *[*]*

[*]Chia seeds

I love adding these tiny yet nutritionally strong seeds to my breakfast. Rich in omega-3s, more calcium by weight than milk and a complete protein, they can easily be used as an egg substitute or as a thickener. It's no wonder the word 'chia' means 'strength' in Mayan!

[*]Ground flaxseeds

I consider flaxseeds to be a 'superfood', but to benefit from their high concentration of polyphenols and omega-3s, they have to be ground down. Sprinkle onto breakfast bowls, throw into smoothies, add to burger or baking mixes or use as a replacement for breadcrumb coatings.

'Superfood' powders:

- **[*]Matcha:** a glorious green powder with amazing nutritional powers. I love taking the time to traditionally prepare and drink this – the euphoric sensation of mental alertness and deep relaxation feels like meditation. The release of caffeine is slowed, stimulating alertness and inducing relaxation, without the characteristic crash in energy. And matcha has been shown to improve attention, reaction times and memory.

- [*]**Maca powder:** has a distinct, earthy flavour – malt-like and slightly butterscotchy – so I tend not to use too much in one go, and fortunately only a small amount is needed to reap the benefits. Packed with vitamins and minerals, it is also a good vegan source of iron as one 5g teaspoon provides almost 5–10 per cent of the RDA for adults.
- [*]**Cacao powder:** the source of everything chocolate-based, cacao is a powerhouse of nutrition. 'Cacao' refers to foods derived from the whole cacao bean that has remained 'raw' and unroasted, whereas 'cocoa' indicates foods made from roasted beans, usually accompanied by sugars, fats, hydrogenated oils, E-numbers, artificial flavours and dairy. Just 20g of dark chocolate every three days lowers CRP levels, suggesting that cocoa (and cacao with stronger flavanol content) may reduce inflammation.
- [*]**Moringa powder:** this is one of the first medicinal plants I was gifted as a remedy, and although there is no research to back up the anti-arthritis claims, it does have a high nutritional value. An acquired, grass-like and earthy taste, it's suited to boosting the flavour of curries, soups and smoothies.

Note: other 'superfood' powders worth having a try, if you can, include spirulina, açaí, wheatgrass and baobab.

Buckwheat flour

Its name is misleading, as it is not a form of wheat and is completely gluten free. Along with spelt and quinoa, it's an 'ancient grain' and has remained unchanged for hundreds of years. Buckwheat foods help to lower cholesterol and GI levels, while providing more antioxidants and minerals than other grains.

Shiitake mushrooms

With a fortunate extra 'i' in the spelling, these edible Asian forest mushrooms have been cultivated for centuries. They are the second-most popular edible mushrooms globally, but have the number-one spot for nutritional and medicinal value. Consuming shiitake mushrooms daily was shown in one study to improve immunity with a reduction in CRP.

Star anise

Aptly named seeds in star-shaped pods, packed with polyphenols, these can be used whole (simmered in sauces or marinades, but not added too early and removed before serving) or ground to a powder.

Cardamom pods

Cardamom is a small green pod containing tiny black seeds. With a strong and sweet flavour, this can be used whole during cooking (but discarded before eating) or the seeds can be ground.

Cardamom has been found to have strong anti-inflammatory properties.

Garam masala

Variety is the spice of life, and of garam masala. This is an aromatic spice mix, differing in composition regionally across South Asia. Frequently used to give a warm, spicy flavour to Indian curries, it usually includes cumin, cloves, coriander, cinnamon, cardamom, nutmeg and black pepper. As we learned in Chapter 2, black pepper is packed with anti-inflammatory piperine and cinnamaldehyde is the active polyphenolic component of cinnamon. For any unfamiliar spices or herbs, flip back to Chapter 2 (see pp. 32–36).

Hemp seeds

Seeds of the hemp plant ('hemp hearts' with the fibrous shell removed) can easily be eaten raw thrown into sauces or smoothies, or made into hemp seed oil, milk and flour. Hemp is comprised of over 80 per cent of omega fatty acids, and has an optimal omega-3:omega-6 ratio for human health.

Note: buckwheat flour, shiitake mushrooms and hemp seeds are not classified as superfoods, but are often under debate as being so!

Soy (or soya-based foods)

Genistein is *the* major active polyphenolic compound within the soybean, as we learned in Chapter 2 (see p. 36).

- **Tofu:** in a process similar to cheesemaking, tofu is made by pressing and solidifying condensed soya milk into blocks that range from silken (ideal for creamy desserts) to extra firm (perfect for crispy pan frying).
- **Tempeh:** packed with protein, prebiotics and probiotics, tempeh is processed by cooking, then fermenting soybeans and forming them into a block. It has a meaty texture and a nutty, mushroomy flavour.
- **Tamari:** a Japanese version of soy sauce, this is derived from fermented soybeans, but is a wheat-free condiment. Splashed into stir-fries or flavouring sauces, it has a richer and gentler flavour than the saltier Chinese soy sauce.

Polenta

Made by milling corn into a coarse flour with a sweetcorn-yellow colour and sweetness, humble polenta is a great gluten-free alternative that can be cooked with water to form a porridge-like consistency, or left to solidify into a piece that can be cut up and pan-fried, grilled, baked or sautéed. Neutral on the tastebuds, it easily absorbs the flavours of other ingredients.

Jackfruit

Growing in demand by the day in the plant-based world, jackfruit imitates meat well. Two hundred times the weight of a mango, it looks like an oblong cantaloupe melon with spikes. Sounds intimidating? Well, for us Westerners in particular, it is usually sold cut and ready to eat. Unripe, it is perfect for savoury dishes, whereas ripened jackfruit is sticky sweet and ideal for desserts or smoothies. It is packed with healthy antioxidants, including vitamin C, which – as we know from p. 38 – helps to reduce inflammation.

[*]Kale

Kale has acquired superfood status in the last decade, with kale crisps (or chips, for some), smoothies and salads having become fundamental to any health-conscious cook's repertoire. Rich in anti-inflammatory antioxidants, including vitamin C, and vitamin K, it is also high in fibre, so it's good for gut health too. Curly-leaf kale is the most common type and cavolo nero is ideal for crisp making. If purchasing kale in its whole raw form, remove the tough stems running down the centre of the leaves before slicing it up.

Blackstrap molasses

Blackstrap molasses crops up annually as black treacle in bonfire toffee. But rich in iron (initially, I had critically low levels), blackstrap is a traditional natural remedy for anaemia, and while it might sound kooky, some arthritics swear by taking 1–2 tablespoons of it every day.

Nutritional yeast

Let me save you from the mistake I made by telling you now that 'easy-bake yeast' is not the same as nutritional yeast. Defined in the Urban Dictionary as 'vegan crack', it is used in many dairy-free savoury dishes. If dairy could be the 'trigger' food for your arthritis, then this is the ideal substitute.

Brown rice

Brown rice retains the nutrients that refined white rice lacks such as vitamins, minerals and phytonutrients, has a lower GI and is completely worth the extra 10 to 15 minutes' cooking time.

To prepare, measure 70–90g per person and rinse in a sieve under cold running water. Bring 2.5 to 3 litres of water to the boil in a large pot (with an accompanying lid). Add the rice to the water and stir with a sprinkle of salt, then boil uncovered for 28–30 minutes. Drain the rice for about 15 seconds before returning to the pot and covering with the lid for 5–10 minutes of steam time, then fluff through with a fork. You can find brown rice in numerous recipes in Chapter 5.

[*]Quinoa

It took a while for me to pronounce this word correctly ('keen-waa'). It looks similar to couscous, and it's available in red, white or black. Gluten-free, it has a high nutritional value, including the perfect balance of all nine essential amino acids, making it a complete protein. It can be stirred into salads or served as a side.

Kefir

Kefir is a probiotic and fermented-milk beverage with anti-inflammatory, antioxidant and antimicrobial properties, as well as supporting the immune system. Kefir may also be made using non-dairy, plant-based alternatives. As kefir is fermented, it has a much lower lactose content and is like a drinkable yoghurt.

Arthritis Foodie Planning

Whether you want to go fully Arthritis Foodie, or you just need a bit of help in experimenting, I would recommend trying it for 6 to 12 weeks before reintroducing any potential trigger and inflammatory foods into your routine. If you consider that medication takes a minimum of 12 weeks to make any noticeable changes, then this makes sense. As with anything, it takes time, and although you may not see any outer visible changes, on the inside your gut bugs might be dancing and singing! As well as your arthritis symptoms, track how you are feeling – in both body and mind – as you try new recipes, exercises, sleep hygiene and mental wellbeing tips (see Chapters 7, 8 and 9, respectively), using the 'Trigger Tracker' on p. 82.

Cooking tips

- Keep your store-cupboard and fridge stocked with essentials, as listed in this chapter.
- Plan recipes for the week ahead, so you feel calm in knowing what you will be eating, and pre-make any sauces and salad dressings if you will be using them frequently in the week.
- Get your friends and family to help. This makes the process more enjoyable, as well as being a support for you on your bad days.

- Measure out the ingredients and do any prep with them before starting to cook. If you have time to do this, it will be a much more relaxing way to cook.
- Use pre-peeled and pre-cut vegetables (or frozen) if you are struggling to prepare fresh ones.
- Sit down to chop, rather than standing at your worktop for long periods.
- Bulk/batch cook where you can, so that you can eat during the week and freeze some for when you do not really feel up to cooking.
- Put music on while you work and see it as mindfulness and time for yourself – enjoy the process.
- Moderation is okay. Don't worry if you 'fall off the wagon', but track it, and remember the 80/20 rule (see p. 5) and the fire and water analogy (see p. 48).
- Use kitchen gadget aids (see p. 68) whenever you feel you need them.
- As there is a changeover in eating habits, you will need a change of drinking habits too. As well as a reducing alcohol, you will likely need to boost the amount of water you drink daily because of the increased intake of fibrous foods. I try to drink 2–3 litres a day.

Trigger Tracker Template

Rheumatologist Lauren Freid encourages her patients to keep journals, tracking food intake alongside arthritis symptoms of pain, stiffness, swelling and fatigue. It's a great way to identify patterns and dietary triggers that may be worsening your arthritis. Many people can be sensitive to dairy or gluten, for instance, but not everyone has the same trigger. The only way to know is to do the work, so you can potentially avoid flares of pain, choosing the foods that work for your body and arthritis. Putting in the time now to become informed allows you to make healthier choices in the future – and making these choices will eventually become second nature. It is important to remember that food is medicine for the mind, body and soul.

Working with a dietitian or nutritionist to help with this process may be beneficial too. I would recommend recording how you feel the day after – i.e. reflecting on what you ate and did activity-wise the previous day. Once you have completed 12 weeks, and tracked any significant changes, repeat the process, using anything you have already learned (e.g. patterns and triggers).

Week 1
Cut out all potential triggers and inflammatory substances, as listed in Chapter 3.
Weeks 2–6
Continue with cutting out inflammatory foods.
Week 7
Reintroduce one 'inflammatory' item and review, noting the effects.
Week 8
Reintroduce one new 'inflammatory' item and review.
Week 9
Reintroduce 1–2 new 'inflammatory' items and review.
Week 10
Reintroduce 1–2 more new 'inflammatory' items and review.
Week 11
Reintroduce 1–3 more new 'inflammatory' items and review.
Week 12
Reintroduce 1–4 more new 'inflammatory' items and review.

Use a scale of 1–10 to rate reactions, where 0 is extremely good and 10 is very poor.

Here are two example entries:

Entry 1:
Week/date
Week 6
05.04.2020
Breakfast
Porridge with oat milk, banana, chia seeds and honey
Lunch
Mushroom soup
Dinner
Chickpea burgers, salad, and sweet-potato wedges with tomato salsa
Drinks
• Matcha
• Green tea with lemon
• Peppermint tea
• Water
Snacks
• Brazil nuts and raisins
• Peach
Stress and mindfulness (1–10)
4
Exercise (1–10)
5, long walk
Sleep (1–10)
1, good sleep
How do you feel today – pain levels, gut health, swelling, symptoms? (1–10)

2, minimal pain levels
Any potential triggers today? New inflammatory substance introduction?
No
Entry 2:
Week/date
Week 10
01.05.2020
Breakfast
Chocolate smoothie bowl
Lunch
Harissa lentil pot
Dinner
Pizza with chorizo
Drinks
• Water
Snacks
• Spiced nuts
Stress and mindfulness (1–10)
4
Exercise (1–10)
7, light yoga and a walk
Sleep (1–10)
6
How do you feel today – pain levels, gut health, swelling, symptoms? (1–10)
8
Any potential triggers today? New inflammatory substance introduction?
Processed meat (new), gluten and dairy (new)

5

Your 65 Tried-and-True Recipes

'A recipe has no soul; you as the cook must bring soul to the recipe.'
Thomas Keller, Michelin-starred chef, restaurateur, author

I give you your 65 recipes to supercharge your health for the better. Before using a recipe, please refer to the following information and tips:

- **Sea salt (Himalayan) and black pepper:** unless otherwise stated, this is to taste; usually a 'twist' or two of the mills will suffice
- **Plant milk:** almond, soya, hemp seed, oat, coconut, cashew, brown rice, hazelnut and tigernut
- **Olive oil:** all oil used in these recipes is extra virgin olive oil, unless otherwise stated
- **Eggs, meat, vegetables and fish:** all organic, where possible
- **Grating:** use the grater setting on your food processor, or ask for help
- **V, Veg, DF, GF:** these denote vegan, vegetarian, dairy free and gluten free, respectively (or the option to be)
- **Vegan alternative to honey:** use maple syrup, agave or date syrup

- **Vegan alternative to eggs:** use a chia egg recipe (1 tablespoon chia or ground flaxseeds with 2½ tablespoons water and 10 minutes rest time).
- **For any shop-bought products:** tomato purée, mayonnaise, wholegrain mustard, apple cider vinegar, oils, nut butters, vegetable stocks, choose 100 per cent wholefood and organic
- **Apple cider vinegar:** make sure it is 'with the mother' (this means it's unfiltered and unrefined, with beneficial bacteria, yeast and protein)
- **For dried fruits:** choose sulphite-free and organic (apricots will be brown not orange!)
- **Tinned coconut milk:** Chakoah is the best brand I've found
- **Flour-based recipes:** I mainly use brown rice flour or buckwheat flour, but other GF options include oat, almond and coconut
- **Pasta:** in general use GF versions (e.g. red lentil)
- **Rice noodles:** the best brand I have found is King Soba organic brown rice and wakame noodles; but white rice vermicelli noodles may be more accessible
- **Roasted garlic:** cook in the oven unpeeled for 10 minutes on 190–200°C, then cool and peel
- **For oven-based recipes:** the temperature is based on a °C fan-based oven, so you may need to adjust accordingly. See the conversion table on page 319–320.

Your 65 Tried-and-True Recipes

Note: all recipes marked 'V' are either intrinsically vegan or can be made vegan using substitutes (e.g. maple syrup for honey, chia or flaxseeds for eggs).

Breakfast

- Perfect Porridge
- Morning Matcha Smoothie
- Raspberry Ripple Pancakes
- Blueberry Chia Pot
- Chocolate Smoothie Bowl
- Strawberry Layered Oats
- Breakfast Sweet Muffins
- Spicy Baked Beans
- Plant-based Breakfast
- Chorizo-flavoured Shakshuka

Small plates

- Warming Parsnip Soup
- Creamy Mushroom Soup (Hold the Cream)
- Polyphenol Cauli-power
- Crispy Kale, Three Ways
- Courgette and Carrot Fritters
- Sweet, Spicy Sprouts
- Rainbow Buddha Bowl with Tahini Dressing
- Charred Broccoli and Turmeric Cream

Large plates

- Tempeh Sri Lankan Fried Rice
- Cashew Cream Pasta
- Satay Salmon (or Tofu)
- Multiple Mushroom Risotto
- Raspberry Sauce Salad
- Shroomballs and Sauce
- Cajun Salmon Burgers
- Butter-bean Squash Salad with Indulgent Sesame Sauce
- Chickpea Burgers
- BBQ Sticky Rice
- Mum's Easy Salmon Stir-fry with Noodles
- Korma-style Curry
- Basil Emily Salad
- Kidney Bean Falafels
- Victoria's Gut-healing Bone Broth
- Harissa Lentil Pot
- Thai Green Curry

Desserts, snacks and treats

- Sweet and Curry-spiced Mixed Nuts
- Cacao-dusted 'Truffles'
- Raspberry and Peanut Flapjacks
- Raspberry Vegan 'Cheese' Cake
- Bright Blueberry Muffins
- Soft Banana Bread
- Choco-avo-late Mousse
- Vegan Mango Lassi

- Baked and Spiced Chickpeas
- Fudgy Sweet-potato Brownies
- Deconstructed Pear Crumble
- Dad's Essential-mineral-fuelled Snack

Drinks, juices and smoothies

- Matcha Moment
- Nausea-knocking Peppermint Tea
- Chocolate M*lk Shake
- Ginger Kick (Banana, Mango, Ginger)
- Strawberries and 'Cream'
- Pecan Pie Shake
- Mango and Raspberry Refresher
- Maca Smoothie
- Indulgent Hot Cacao
- Berry Power
- Warming Chai

Sauces, sides and dips

- Cooling Mint Yoghurt Dip
- Butter-bean Burger Sauce
- Tomato Relish Sauce
- Homemade Coleslaw
- Basil Salad Dressing
- Hummus
- Tahini Salad Dressing

Breakfast

Perfect Porridge

V, Veg, DF, GF

Porridge is my go-to breakfast, especially in the colder months of the year. It is warming, keeps you feeling full with a slow release of energy and can be topped with almost anything.

SERVES 1

Ingredients

40g whole rolled oats
150ml plant milk
100ml water
1 tbsp chia seeds or flaxseeds
Toppings: dried fruit and seeds; fresh fruit; nut butter; honey (or a vegan alternative – see p. 85)

Steps

- Pour the oats into a pan and stir in your plant milk and water.
- Place it on a high heat until it starts to lightly bubble in 2 minutes, then reduce the heat straight away to a low–medium simmer and stir.
- Stir occasionally for 5–6 minutes, until all of the loose liquid has been absorbed, and the porridge has a thick and creamy consistency.
- Remove from the heat and let it stand for 3 minutes to cool, adding the toppings of your choice before eating.

Morning Matcha Smoothie

V, Veg, DF, GF

We will come on to how to make a matcha latte on p. 153, but if you would like to get your matcha fix a different way, then there's this.

SERVES 1

Ingredients

1 banana
40g whole rolled oats
200ml plant milk
½ tsp honey (optional; or a vegan alternative – see p. 85)
1–2 tbsp water
½ tsp matcha powder
Ice cubes (optional)

Steps

- Blend the banana, oats, plant milk and honey (if using).
- Add in the matcha mix – see 'Matcha Moment', p. 153, for detailed instructions, or if you are using a lower grade of matcha, simply add it straight in.
- Blend with ice (optional) and serve.

Raspberry Ripple Pancakes

V, Veg, DF, GF

These are a scrumptious weekend treat that the whole family (or just you) can enjoy. I always have containers of frozen fruit in the freezer at the ready for using in recipes like this one.

MAKES 4

Ingredients

For the pancake batter:

Pinch of ground cinnamon
½ tsp baking powder
150g buckwheat flour
1 tsp coconut sugar
200ml plant milk
1 large egg, whisked (or an egg substitute – see p. 86)
Coconut oil for frying

For the raspberry coulis:

150g frozen raspberries
2 tbsp water
2 tbsp honey (or a vegan alternative – see p. 85)
8 tbsp coconut yoghurt

Steps

- Fill a large mixing bowl with all of the dry ingredients and mix well.
- Slowly pour in the plant milk before adding the egg (or egg substitute) and combine well.

- Place your raspberries into a pan and cook on a low–medium heat while you start to make the pancakes (around 20 minutes).
- Heat the coconut oil in a small frying pan and cook the pancake mixture, a ladleful at a time, for 1–2 minutes on each side. Pile the pancakes on to a plate as you cook them and keep them warm.
- Keep stirring the coulis while you cook the pancakes, and when it starts to thicken add the water and the honey.
- Cut the pile of pancakes into quarters like slices of cake, or serve them individually, topped with your raspberry coulis and coconut yoghurt.

Blueberry Chia Pot

V, Veg, DF, GF

A really simple recipe to make ahead, so that you can grab and go, saving time in the morning. I usually make this kind of overnight recipe in a jar.

SERVES 1

Ingredients

200ml plant milk
4 tbsp chia seeds
2 tbsp whole rolled oats
2 tbsp blueberries
1 tsp honey (or a vegan alternative – see p. 85)
Sunflower or pumpkin seeds, to serve (optional)

Steps

- Fill a glass or a jar with the plant milk, then add the chia seeds and oats. Stir well.
- Leave in the fridge overnight.
- Top with the blueberries and the honey in the morning; you could also add sunflower or pumpkin seeds.

Chocolate Smoothie Bowl

V, Veg, DF, GF

Another healthy-yet-feels-like-a-treat kind of breakfast, this smoothie bowl is delicious in the summer, and could even be used as a fruity, nutty dessert – say, as an alternative to rice pudding.

SERVES 2

Ingredients

1 banana
1 avocado
150ml plant milk
1½ tbsp maca powder
1 tbsp raw cacao powder
3 tbsp whole rolled oats
2 tbsp mixed nuts (almonds, walnuts, pecans)
2 tbsp date syrup
Toppings: 2 tbsp granola, fresh fruit

Steps

- Blend all of the above together until smooth, then top with the granola and fresh fruit of your choice.

Strawberry Layered Oats

V, Veg, DF, GF

A scrumptious summer breakfast recipe: overnight oats, layered with strawberries. In the summer, it may be too hot for hot porridge, so the solution is overnight oats!

SERVES 1

Ingredients
4 large strawberries
40g whole rolled oats
1 tbsp chia seeds
1 tbsp ground flaxseeds (optional)
200ml plant milk
50ml water
2 tsp honey (or maple syrup)
Extra strawberries

Steps

- Chop up the 4 strawberries and place in a glass or a jar.
- Add the oats, chia seeds, flaxseeds (if using), plant milk, water and honey or maple syrup.
- Stir well and leave in the fridge overnight.
- Top in the morning with extra strawberries.

Breakfast Sweet Muffins

Veg, DF, GF

Oats, bananas, nuts and apples – the perfect combination in a warm muffin, baked for the morning or for eating during the week.

MAKES 12

Ingredients

Dry ingredients:

100g whole rolled oats
40g pumpkin seeds
100g brown rice flour
75g chopped dates
1 tsp baking powder
2 tsp ground cinnamon
½ tsp ground nutmeg
1 tsp ground ginger
Sea salt
Coconut sugar – to top

Wet ingredients:

1 egg
2 tbsp melted coconut oil
6 tbsp honey (or a vegan alternative – see p. 85)
100ml plant milk
3 mashed bananas
2 small apples, unpeeled and grated

Steps

- Mix together all the dry ingredients in a large bowl and set aside.
- Whisk the egg, oil and honey and then blend in the milk.
- Fold the wet ingredients into the dry ingredients and, when almost combined, add the mashed bananas and grated apples.
- Do not overmix. Just stir until the fruit is evenly distributed, then spoon into the holes of a greased muffin tin tray (about 2 tablespoons per muffin).
- Sprinkle a pinch of coconut sugar on to each muffin before placing in the oven.
- Bake at 180°C for 30–35 minutes, until golden brown, then remove from the oven and leave to cool and set for 15–20 minutes.
- Store in an airtight container in the fridge for 3–4 days.

Spicy Baked Beans

V, Veg, DF, GF

Baked beans used to be my staple favourite, and this is an easy alternative recipe to make at home. You could add them to a slice of sourdough. Yum!

SERVES 2

Ingredients

1 bell pepper
1 courgette
2 garlic cloves, finely chopped

½ tbsp oil
1 tsp chilli flakes (optional)
½ tsp paprika
½ tsp cayenne pepper
1 tsp dried harissa spices
1 tin cannellini beans
2 tsp tomato purée
3 tbsp plant milk
Sea salt and black pepper

Steps

- Chop the pepper and courgette into small chunks.
- Cook the garlic and pepper in a pan with the oil on a medium heat for 5 minutes, then add the courgette, followed by the spices, sea salt and black pepper.
- Add the cannellini beans and stir well.
- Add the tomato purée and plant milk, and reduce the heat to thicken.

Plant-based Breakfast

V, Veg, DF, GF

A different approach to the usual breakfast 'fry-up', but in this case there is no deep frying of processed meats, featuring the shiitake mushroom instead.

SERVES 2

Ingredients
2 sweet potatoes
Olive oil, for drizzling, cooking

120g shiitake mushrooms
2 jubilee vine tomatoes/large salad tomatoes
1 avocado
2 eggs (V: lightly fry some firm tofu, cut into cubes)
¼ tsp dried oregano
50ml plant milk
1 tsp apple cider vinegar
5g chives, chopped
1 tsp mayonnaise (or vegan mayo)
200g spinach
Sea salt and black pepper

Steps

- Preheat the oven to 180°C. Peel the sweet potato and dice into small cubes of around 1–2cm. Place on a baking tray with a drizzle of olive oil, sea salt and black pepper. Place in the oven for 25–30 minutes, turning halfway through.
- Meanwhile, cut the mushrooms into chunks, the tomatoes into halves and the avocado into slices.
- Griddle the mushrooms and tomatoes for 3–5 minutes, on a low–medium heat with olive oil, sea salt and black pepper.
- Whisk together the eggs, oregano and the plant milk, and add to an oiled hot saucepan to make scrambled eggs. Stir until fluffy, should take 3–5 minutes, so only do these two steps when the potatoes are almost ready. If vegan, lightly fry your tofu at this point.
- Place the cooked sweet potatoes in a bowl with the apple cider vinegar, chives and mayonnaise.
- Plate everything up and add the spinach raw to the plate (or lightly cook if you prefer).

Chorizo-flavoured Shakshuka

Veg, DF, GF

Recreating the smoky flavour of chorizo without the chorizo – and it adds such a tasty flavour to this recipe. So scrumptious to dip with sourdough bread.

SERVES 2

Ingredients
4 large eggs
For the vegetables:
3 garlic cloves
1 red onion
1 bell pepper
200g mushrooms
1 tbsp olive oil
2 x 400g tins chopped tomatoes
1 tbsp tomato purée
1 x 400g tin butter beans, drained
Sea salt and black pepper
Handful of fresh coriander leaves
For the spice mixture:
½ tsp chilli flakes/powder
2 tsp smoked paprika
½ tsp ground cumin
½ tsp garlic granules
½ tsp onion granules
½ tsp ground coriander
¼ tsp ground nutmeg

1 tsp paprika
1 tbsp olive oil

Steps

- Prepare the spice mixture in a small bowl and set aside.
- Peel and chop the garlic, red onion, pepper and mushrooms.
- Fry the garlic and onion together in the oil in a large pan (one that has a lid) for 3 minutes.
- Add the pepper and cook for 5 minutes before adding the mushrooms. Fry for 2–3 minutes before adding the tinned tomatoes, tomato purée, spice mixture and salt and pepper, then simmer for 10 minutes until it all thickens.
- Stir in the butter beans then use the back of a spoon to make 4 wells in the pan mixture, adding an egg to each well using ramekins to drop them in. Cover with a lid for 5 minutes until the eggs are cooked.
- Serve garnished with fresh coriander and dipping breads on the side.

Small Plates

Warming Parsnip Soup

V, Veg, DF, GF

Parsnips are often forgotten about when it's not Sunday-roast time, but, they're a versatile vegetable with a sweet and moreish flavour.

SERVES 2

Ingredients

6–8 parsnips (around 800g)
½ tsp black pepper
½ tsp sea salt
3 garlic cloves
1 large white onion
1 tbsp olive oil, plus extra for drizzling
½ tsp thyme
½ tsp rosemary
500ml hot water
1 cube vegetable stock
200ml plant milk
1 tsp balsamic vinegar

Steps

- Preheat the oven to 200°C. Peel and chop the parsnips into small chunks, then place on a baking tray with a drizzle of olive oil, ½ tsp black pepper and ½ tsp sea salt. Cook for 25 minutes.

- While the parsnips are cooking, peel and chop the garlic and onion. Slowly soften in a pan with the olive oil for 10 minutes on a low–medium heat, being careful not to singe or burn them.
- Add the roasted parsnips, thyme and rosemary and lightly heat together for 2–3 minutes, before adding the hot water and vegetable stock.
- Simmer for 20 minutes, then add the plant milk and balsamic vinegar and blend until smooth.

Creamy Mushroom Soup (Hold the Cream)

V, Veg, DF, GF

When I first started cooking, this was one of the first recipes my friend Mahi fell in love with and now makes frequently – probably more than I do! It's creamy, without any dairy.

SERVES 4

Ingredients

4 red onions, peeled and finely chopped
3 garlic cloves, peeled and finely chopped
2 tbsp olive oil
900g mixed mushrooms: 350g closed-cup, 350g chestnut, 200g portobello, roughly chopped
5 sticks celery, chopped (optional)
100g walnuts (optional), roughly chopped
1.2 litres water
1 vegetable stock cube
1 tbsp honey (or maple syrup)
1 tbsp balsamic vinegar
Sea salt and black pepper

Steps

- Cook the onions and garlic in a large pan with the olive oil and after 5 minutes add the mushrooms, celery and walnuts (if using). Add the salt and pepper.
- After another 5 minutes, add the water and wait until it is bubbling before adding the vegetable stock cube. Stir well.
- Simmer on a low heat for 40–60 minutes to thicken, partially covered with the pan lid.
- Blend in a food processor with the honey or maple syrup and balsamic vinegar.

Polyphenol Cauli-power

V, Veg, DF, GF

This is my go-to dish when I'm feeling under the weather: warming, spicy and full of phytochemicals in the form of aromatic spices. You could have it on its own or with my Cooling Mint Yoghurt Dip (see p. 175).

SERVES 2

Ingredients

1 cauliflower

For the spices:

½ tsp ground coriander

½ tsp chilli flakes

½ tsp turmeric

½ tsp ground cinnamon

½ tsp garam masala

2 tbsp olive oil

Sea salt and black pepper

To serve:
2 tsp lime juice
Fresh coriander

Steps

- Preheat the oven to 190°C.
- Stir all the spice ingredients together in a small bowl.
- Separate the cauliflower into chunks, using the natural shape and size of the florets. Place in a large bowl and pour the spice mixture all over, plus the oil, stirring well until all covered.
- You can marinate the cauliflower if you have the time; if not, throw on to a baking parchment-covered baking tray. Roast for 25 minutes until tender, rolling the cauliflower around halfway through the cooking time.
- Drizzle with the fresh lime juice, then top with coriander. Serve with the mint yoghurt dip, if desired.

Crispy Kale, Three Ways

V, Veg, DF, GF

Crispy kale, as a side dish or as a snack – I eat them like crisps! You can flavour kale crisps in a variety of ways, and here are three of my favourites.

SERVES 2

Ingredients
100g curly leaf kale
½–1 tsp olive oil
Hot chilli and garlic:

½ tsp chilli flakes (add more if you can handle it!)
1 tsp garlic granules
Sea salt and black pepper
Onion and chive:
1 tsp onion granules
4 tsp (20g) chopped fresh chives
Sea salt and black pepper
Pecan maple:
100g whole or chopped pecans
1 tsp maple syrup
Sea salt and black pepper

Steps

- Preheat the oven for 5 minutes at 180°C.
- Place the kale on a baking tray with olive oil (taking care not to drown it) and your chosen toppings.
- Bake for 5 minutes, turning halfway through – it may need longer or less, depending on the strength of your oven.
- My advice – watch the kale and don't leave it alone, as it's quick to burn (had plenty of mishaps over the last few years).

Courgette and Carrot Fritters

Veg, DF, GF
One for the lunch box. Really easy to make, and they store well too.

MAKES 6

Ingredients
4 carrots (350g)
2 courgettes

60g brown rice flour
30g flaxseeds
1 egg
¼ tsp smoked paprika
½ tsp garlic granules or 1 garlic clove, grated
½ tsp chilli flakes (optional)
Olive oil, for frying
Sea salt and black pepper

Steps

- Grate the carrots in a food processor and place on a tea towel, scoop together and squeeze out the liquid over the sink then place in a large mixing bowl. This is an important step, so please do not skip.
- Repeat the above step with the courgettes and add both to the mixing bowl.
- Whisk the egg and add into the bowl, mix well.
- Add all of the remaining ingredients, stir well until fully combined.
- Heat a drizzle of olive oil in a pan. Once hot scoop a spoonful of mixture into the pan and pat into a patty fritter shape using the back of a spatula. Cook a few at a time if you have the room in your pan.
- Cook for 3–4 minutes on each side on a medium high heat, so as not to burn, but cook to a crisp.
- Serve straight away with or leave to cool and store for lunches.

Sweet, Spicy Sprouts

V, Veg, DF, GF

Why would anyone choose to eat this unwanted Christmas vegetable? Well, I decided to forget any preconceived ideas I had about this unloved vegetable and began to experiment. It's now a favourite in our household.

SERVES 4

Ingredients

500g Brussels sprouts
2 tbsp honey or maple syrup
1 tsp chilli flakes
2 tsp olive oil
Sea salt and black pepper
30g flaked almonds (optional), to serve

Steps

- Preheat the oven to 200°C. Prepare the sprouts, leaving them whole.
- Grab a deep oven dish or oven baking tray and throw in the sprouts with the honey or maple syrup, chilli flakes, olive oil, sea salt and black pepper. Toss around until they're all fully coated.
- Place them in the oven to bake for 20–30 minutes, or until the sprouts are lightly charred and crisp on the outside and toasted on the bottoms.
- Sprinkle the flaked almonds over them before serving, if desired. Sweet, salty, delicious!

Rainbow Buddha Bowl with Tahini Dressing

V, Veg, DF, GF

A deliciously refreshing salad. You can play about with the colours and experiment with your chosen vegetable, depending on the season.

SERVES 2

Ingredients

80g quinoa
100g radishes, trimmed
2 large vine tomatoes
120g strawberries (hulled) or cherries
½ yellow pepper
30g rocket leaves
1 carrot
1 large avocado
1 x 400g tin butter beans, drained and rinsed
Sesame seeds, to sprinkle
Wedge of lime, to garnish
To serve:
Tahini Salad Dressing (see p. 166)

Steps

- Rinse the quinoa before cooking and place in a pan of salted boiling water on a medium heat for 15–20 minutes or until tender. Rinse, then cool.

- Slice the radishes, tomatoes, strawberries or cherries and pepper, and distribute evenly between 2 bowls. Add a handful of rocket leaves to each bowl.
- Peel and grate the carrot, then add.
- Halve the avocado, adding one half to each bowl, then add the butter beans, distributing proportionately.
- Add the cooked quinoa, sprinkle with sesame seeds and pour over the tahini dressing, then garnish with a wedge of lime (to squeeze before eating!).

Charred Broccoli and Turmeric Cream

V, Veg, DF, GF

Inspired by a couple of plant-based restaurants I have visited, I wanted to create this flavour-packed dish with key anti-inflammatory properties in mind.

SERVES 2

Ingredients
1 whole broccoli head
¼ tsp salt
Olive oil, for drizzling
For the turmeric cream:
175g hemp seeds or cashew nuts
25ml apple cider vinegar
100ml plant milk
¼ tsp ground turmeric
1 tsp honey (or a vegan alternative – see p. 85)
Sea salt and black pepper

Steps

- For the turmeric cream, soak the hemp seeds or cashew nuts in warm water for 25 minutes.
- Preheat the grill until hot. Place the broccoli in a bowl of boiling salted water for 5 minutes, then drain and rinse in cold water.
- Season the broccoli with salt and pepper, drizzle with oil and grill on a baking tray until the broccoli is charred, for 7–10 minutes on each side.
- In the final 5 minutes of the broccoli's cooking time, strain the hemp seeds or cashew nuts and place in a blender with the apple cider vinegar, plant milk, turmeric, honey and a sprinkle of salt. Blend until smooth.
- Serve the broccoli with the turmeric cream sauce drizzled on top.

Large Plates

Tempeh Sri Lankan Fried Rice

Veg, DF, GF

Recreating a classic takeaway dish that my sister loves, this is a fusion of flavours and can be served with tempeh or egg or chicken.

SERVES 2

Ingredients

Either 2 chicken breasts or 1 x 200g pack tempeh
150g brown rice
Sesame oil, for drizzling
2 eggs, beaten (optional – leave out if vegan)
For the stir-fry vegetables:
1 garlic clove
1 red chilli, deseeded
1 red onion
1 bell pepper
200g mushrooms
1 large carrot, grated
150g beansprouts
For the sauce:
2 garlic cloves, chopped
Seeds from 2 cardamom pods, crushed or powdered
½ tsp ground turmeric
½ tsp ground cinnamon

½ tsp ground ginger
2 tbsp sesame oil
1 tbsp tamari
½ tsp honey (or a vegan alternative – see p. 85)
Sea salt and black pepper
To serve:
20g cashew nuts, chopped
4 spring onions, chopped

Steps

- Mix the sauce ingredients together in a small bowl.
- Chop the chicken or the tempeh into bite-sized chunks. Prepare and chop the stir-fry vegetables.
- Rinse the brown rice and cook using the instructions on p. 88.
- Heat a drizzle of sesame oil in a wok or large frying pan and fry the chicken or tempeh for 7–10 minutes, tossing until fully cooked through. Remove from the wok and set aside.
- Add another drizzle of oil, the garlic, chilli and onion to the wok, cooking for around 5 minutes until softened.
- Slowly add the rest of the vegetables and toss until cooked.
- Drain and add in the cooked brown rice, then make a well in the middle of the pan and add the beaten eggs (if using). Lower the heat to cook the eggs.
- Once the eggs are cooked, slice and separate them into pieces and mix through the rice and vegetables.
- Add the chicken or tempeh back into the pan and cook together for 1–2 minutes before stirring in the sauce.
- Serve garnished with spring onions and cashew nuts.

Cashew Cream Pasta

V, Veg, DF, GF

A creamy pasta dish that you can flavour in numerous ways. This one is garlic and mushroom, but you could also use the chorizo spices from the Chorizo-flavoured Shakshuka (see p. 100).

SERVES 2

Ingredients

155g cashew nuts
2 garlic cloves
1 red onion
1 courgette
250g closed-cup mushrooms
1 tsp olive oil
150g red lentil penne pasta
200ml plant milk
½ tsp onion granules
½ tsp garlic granules or paste
½ tsp sea salt
1 tsp black pepper
Handful of fresh basil (optional), to serve

Steps

- Place the cashew nuts in a bowl of lukewarm water, making sure they are all submerged. Leave them to soak for 30 minutes, but if you have longer, soak them for an hour for an extra-creamy consistency.
- Chop the garlic, onion, courgette and mushrooms.

- Halfway through the cashews' soaking time, in a large frying pan, cook the garlic and onions in the olive oil for 5 minutes until softened, then add the courgette and mushrooms.
- In a separate pan, cook the pasta in a pan of boiling water on a medium heat for around 5 minutes (1–2 minutes less than its full cooking time).
- Drain the pasta, then turn down the heat on the vegetables, before draining the cashews (they should weigh 190g after soaking).
- Put the cashews in a blender with the plant milk, onion granules, garlic granules or paste, the sea salt and black pepper and blend to a smooth paste.
- Stir the cashew sauce into the vegetables, along with the drained pasta and mix well for 1–2 minutes. Garnish with fresh basil to serve.

Satay Salmon (or Tofu)

V, Veg, DF, GF

This is an ultimate favourite of mine and it can be made with salmon or tofu. If using tofu, coating it is key for a crispy outer crunch and a soft centre.

SERVES 2

Ingredients

150g brown rice
20g polenta (for tofu only)
2 organic salmon pieces or 2 portions plain or smoked firm tofu (Tofoo is a good brand for consistency)
Sesame oil, for frying and drizzling

For the spice mixture:
½ tsp ground cumin
½ tsp smoked paprika
½ tsp medium curry powder
½ tsp sea salt
½ tsp black pepper
For the stir-fry vegetables:
1 tbsp sesame or coconut oil
2 garlic cloves, chopped
1 thumb-sized piece fresh ginger, chopped
1 red onion, sliced
1 bell pepper, sliced
1 carrot, grated
½ white cabbage, grated or sliced
80g mangetout
1–2 tsp chilli flakes
2 tbsp tamari
3 tbsp peanut butter
2 tbsp honey (or a vegan alternative – see p. 85)
1 tbsp creamed coconut
400ml coconut milk (I like Chaokoh brand)
Sea salt and black pepper
To serve:
Sesame seeds
Fresh coriander

Steps

- Cook the brown rice, using the instructions on p.79.
- If using salmon: preheat the oven to 200°C and place the pieces on a large piece of foil with a drizzle of sesame oil

and the spice mixture, then close up the foil and place on a baking tray and cook for 15–20 minutes.

- If using tofu, mix together the spice mixture with the polenta in a shallow bowl. Cut the tofu into chunky strips and coat in the polenta and spice mixture, then heat a drizzle of sesame oil in a frying pan and fry for 5–7 minutes on each side, until golden brown (exact timing will depend on size and thickness).
- For the vegetables, add 1 tbsp of coconut or sesame oil to a large cooking pan or wok and fry the garlic, ginger and red onion with some salt and pepper.
- After 5 minutes, add the red or green pepper, carrot and white cabbage and cook until they begin to soften before adding the mangetout.
- Add the chilli flakes, tamari, peanut butter, honey, creamed coconut and stir.
- Add the coconut milk and stir well – the sauce should be thick and creamy.
- Top the rice with the vegetable satay mixture, then add the tofu or salmon on top of this. Then sprinkle over sesame seeds and fresh coriander to garnish before serving.

Multiple Mushroom Risotto

V, Veg, DF, GF

Triple mushroom, creamy risotto, with pine nuts, walnuts, lamb's lettuce and basil. A warming dinner that could easily be heated up for lunches during the week.

SERVES 4

Ingredients

1 red onion
2 garlic cloves
400g mixed mushrooms (180g chestnut mushrooms, 80g shiitake, 140g mini portobello – or any other mix)
1 tbsp olive oil, plus a drizzle
1 tsp thyme leaves
1 tsp rosemary leaves
340g brown rice
1 cube vegetable stock, dissolved in 700ml hot water
500ml plant milk plus 500ml water
90g broken walnuts
1 tsp wholegrain mustard
2 heaped tablespoons of nutritional yeast flakes (optional)
2 shallots (optional)
Sea salt and black pepper

To serve:
Fresh basil

Steps

- Slice the red onion and garlic cloves. Slice the mushrooms too, then set aside.
- Place the onion and garlic in a large, wide saucepan with 1 tablespoon of the olive oil, the thyme, rosemary and the salt and pepper. Sauté for 5 minutes.
- Stir the rice through the onion and garlic, then add stock and water, simmering for 15 minutes.

- During this time, place the mushrooms in a large frying pan with a drizzle of olive oil, salt and pepper, and cook on a medium–low heat for 4–7 minutes. Set aside.
- When the rice has been cooking for 15 minutes, add the plant milk and water, the cooked mushrooms and the wholegrain mustard, and simmer for 30 minutes on a low–medium heat, stirring occasionally.
- Stir the walnuts and nutritional yeast into the risotto once it's cooked.
- Garnish with the basil and serve.

Raspberry Sauce Salad

V, Veg, DF, GF

Sweet and savoury is a delicate dance, but this salad combines both the sharp, acidic taste of balsamic with a raspberry sweetness, fresh crispy salad leaves and warm roasted vegetables.

SERVES 8

Ingredients

For roasting:

1 butternut squash
1 small squash (any variety)
1 (cooking) pumpkin
4 garlic cloves, peeled and chopped
3 tbsp olive oil
1 tbsp honey (or a vegan alternative – see p. 96)
1 tsp chipotle flakes or chilli flakes (optional)
Sea salt and black pepper

For the greens:
1 head of broccoli
150g green beans
1 large red onion
100g flaked almonds
200g bag mixed herb and leaf salad
100g spinach

For the dressing:
1 punnet of raspberries
150ml olive oil
2 tbsp organic honey (or a vegan alternative – see p. 85)
3½ tbsp balsamic vinegar
Pinch of sea salt

Additional options:
2 cooked chicken breasts
30g feta cheese

Steps

- Preheat the oven to 200°C. Peel and chop the roasting vegetables and garlic, and place on 3 trays with the olive oil, honey, chipotle flakes, salt and pepper. Roast for 40–45 minutes.
- Chop the broccoli and green beans, boil in a pan of water for 5–7 minutes, then rinse in cold water to preserve their colour and keep them crisp, and place in a large mixing bowl or salad bowl.
- Peel and cut the red onion in half, then again lengthways. Add the onion to the bowl and stir in the flaked almonds, the mixed salad leaves and the spinach.

- Stir the roasted vegetables into the bowl too.
- Place all the dressing ingredients in a blender and blend well, adding honey, salt and pepper to taste. Transfer to a jug.
- Divide the salad between 4 bowls, then add the chicken or feta cheese (if using) on top.
- Drizzle the raspberry salad dressing all over.

Shroomballs and Sauce

V, Veg, DF, GF

As red meat may be a trigger for some arthritis patients, this recipe recreates the typical meatball flavours for a plant-based and vegan alternative. Serve with a traditional tomato pasta sauce. Carrots and celery also go well in this recipe.

SERVES 4

Ingredients

For the shroomballs mixture:

100g quinoa
300g mushrooms
1 tbsp olive oil
20g flaxseeds
15g fresh basil
2 tsp dried Italian herbs (or equal ½ tsp measures of oregano, rosemary, thyme and dried coriander)
100g brown rice flour, plus extra for sprinkling

For the sauce:
1 garlic clove, peeled
2 small red onions
1 tbsp olive oil, plus extra for oiling
1 courgette
1 x 400g tin chopped tomatoes
2 tbsp tomato purée
1 tsp balsamic vinegar
Sea salt and black pepper
Fresh basil

To serve:
320g cooked red lentil penne pasta, spaghetti or sweet-potato wedges

Steps

- Prepare all the vegetables for the sauce, finely slicing everything, but slice the courgette into half-moons.
- Rinse the quinoa, put in a pan of salted boiling water and cook on a medium heat for 15–20 minutes or until tender. Rinse and cool.
- While the quinoa is cooking, chop and fry the mushrooms in the oil for 5–6 minutes.
- Drain the excess liquid from the mushrooms, then process in a blender with the remaining shroomballs ingredients – or you can do this by hand for a rough mixture.
- Sprinkle a flat surface or chopping board with brown rice flour and mould the shroomballs mixture into balls. Set aside.
- Cook the garlic and red onions in a large pan with the olive oil, salt and pepper. Add the chopped tomatoes, tomato purée and balsamic vinegar and simmer over a low heat.

- Oil a shallow frying pan or griddle pan and fry the shroom balls in it for 5–8 minutes. Separately, stir the sliced half-moon courgettes into the sauce.
- Divide the shroom balls into bowls, pour the sauce on top and serve with pasta or sweet potato wedges and fresh basil.

Cajun Salmon Burgers

DF, GF

I'm always experimenting with flavours and it usually starts with a pasta sauce and migrates into other recipes. I experimented to create my own Cajun seasoning for a roasted vegetable pasta, which became the base for these burgers. Serve with the homemade Tomato Relish Sauce (see p. 163).

SERVES 2

Ingredients

For the burgers:

2 salmon fillets, skinned

Cajun seasoning mix:

4 tsp olive oil

1 tsp garlic granules

½ tsp chilli flakes

1 tsp smoked paprika

½ tsp oregano

½ tsp ground cumin

½ tsp thyme

1 tbsp whole rolled oats

1 garlic clove, chopped
1 sprig of fresh coriander, chopped (about ½ tsp)
½ tsp lime juice
Sea salt and pepper
Olive oil, for frying

For the roast vegetables, to serve:
1 sweet potato
Olive oil, for drizzling and frying
½ roasted butternut squash
1 courgette, griddled
2 lime wedges
Tomato Relish Sauce (see p. 163)

Steps

- Preheat the oven to 190°C. For the vegetables, slice the sweet potato into wedges, skin on, drizzle with olive oil, season with salt and pepper and place on a baking tray. Peel and chop the butternut squash into wedges (store the half you are not using in an airtight container in the fridge). Season and place on the baking tray with the sweet potato.
- Roast in the oven for 40 minutes, turning the vegetables halfway through cooking.
- For the burgers, cut the salmon fillets into small chunks (it's easier to do this when it is cold – you can place the salmon in the freezer for 15 minutes to firm it up if needed).
- Chop and blend all the salmon burger ingredients, along with the Cajun seasoning in a food processor, or by hand, until you have a sticky mixture.

- Mould into patty shapes (they don't have to be perfect!), then heat some olive oil (around 1 tablespoon) and cook the burgers for for 5–6 minutes on each side, until firm and hot in the middle.
- Serve with the sweet potato and butternut squash wedges, griddled courgettes, lime wedges, and Tomato Relish Sauce.

Butter-bean Squash Salad with Indulgent Sesame Sauce

V, Veg, DF, GF

Butter beans and butternut squash make the perfect base of this salad, with a bed of green kale, sweet strawberries and an indulgent honey-sesame-tahini sauce.

SERVES 2

Ingredients

1 butternut squash
2 sweet potatoes
Drizzle of olive oil
5 sprigs of fresh rosemary
200g strawberries
250g curly-leaf kale (or cavolo nero)
1 x 400g tin butter beans, drained and rinsed

For the tahini sesame sauce:

3 tbsp (100g) tahini
2 tbsp honey (or a vegan alternative – see p. 85)

1 tbsp apple cider vinegar
1 tbsp sesame oil
2 tbsp olive oil
1 tsp water
½ tsp garlic granules
Pinch of smoked paprika
Squeeze of lemon juice
Sea salt and black pepper

Steps

- Preheat the oven to 190°C. Peel the butternut squash and sweet potatoes and slice into half-moons/wedges.
- Place the wedges in a deep oven tray with the olive oil, salt, pepper and the sprigs of rosemary. Roast for 35–45 minutes, until soft and slightly golden brown.
- While the vegetables are roasting, rinse and slice the strawberries.
- Mix all the sauce ingredients together; do not worry if it separates – just whisk or pour into an empty jar with a lid and shake.
- Just before the roasted vegetables are done, steam the kale by placing in a metal collander with a lid over a pan of hot water, for 3 minutes maximum, then drain.
- Plate up the salad, with the kale at the bottom, then the butternut squash and sweet potatoes, then the butter beans, the strawberries and a drizzle of the sauce.

Chickpea Burgers

V, Veg, DF, GF

This is effectively all the flavours of hummus, recreated in a burger patty.

MAKES 6 BURGERS

Ingredients

2 x 400g tins chickpeas, drained
2 garlic cloves, peeled
2 spring onions
1 tsp ground cumin
4 tbsp brown rice flour
½ tsp smoked paprika
1 tbsp tahini
1 tsp olive oil, plus extra for frying
Squeeze of lemon juice
Sesame seeds
Sea salt and black pepper
To serve:
Sweet potato wedges
Tomato Relish Sauce (see p.163)
Side salad of choice

Steps

- Smash the chickpeas in a large mixing bowl with a fork or the back of a spoon.
- Chop the garlic and spring onions, and add to the chickpeas.

- Add the remaining ingredients, apart from the sesame seeds and season with salt and pepper.
- Fill a shallow bowl with sesame seeds. Mould your patties with your hands and roll the patties in the sesame seeds to coat them.
- Preheat the oven to 190°C. Bake the burgers for 20–25 minutes on a baking tray lined with baking parchment (or fry for 3–4 minutes on each side).
- Serve with baked sweet potato wedges, and Tomato Relish Sauce (see p.163).

BBQ Sticky Rice

V, Veg, DF, GF

Delicious flavours of BBQ sauce, homemade from your kitchen! You can marinate the tofu, fish or meat if you like, or add them in as they are.

SERVES 2

Ingredients

160g brown rice
1 x 280g packet firm tofu (Tofoo is my favourite)
1 red onion
1 bell pepper, deseeded
1 courgette
Sea salt and black pepper
1 tbsp olive oil

To serve:

Fresh coriander
Homemade Coleslaw (see p. 164)

For the BBQ marinade
1 tsp smoked paprika
1 tbsp honey (or a vegan alternative – see p. 85)
1 tbsp molasses
2 tsp garlic paste
½ tsp Tabasco or chilli powder
1 tsp onion granules
½ tsp dried rosemary
½ tsp ground coriander
½ tsp dried oregano
1 tbsp olive oil
Sea salt and black pepper

Steps

- Cook the brown rice according to the instructions on p. 88.
- Drain and slice the tofu into cubes.
- Mix all the BBQ marinade ingredients in a bowl, then stir in the tofu cubes. There will be more sauce than tofu – this is supposed to happen! Set aside for at least 20 minutes, or if you have time to marinate overnight, better still.
- Peel and chop the red onion and slice the pepper and courgette.
- Ten minutes before the end of the rice cooking time, heat the olive oil in a large pan and fry the onion and pepper, then add the the courgette and finally the tofu, with the marinade.
- Add the brown rice to the pan – it should soak up the BBQ marinade and become sticky.
- Serve with fresh coriander leaves and your slaw.

Mum's Easy Salmon Stir-fry with Noodles

V, Veg, DF, GF

A recipe Mum loves to make at home, usually with salmon that she marinates beforehand, but it also works well with prawns, chicken or tofu too.

SERVES 4

Ingredients
4 keta salmon fillets
Sesame oil for stir-frying
250g brown/rice noodles

For the marinade:
4 tbsp tamari
1 thumb-sized piece fresh ginger (about 5cm), peeled and grated
1 garlic clove, crushed
4 tsp honey (or a vegan alternative – see p. 85)
Juice of ½ lime, plus extra for squeezing
Sea salt and black pepper

Stir-fry vegetable suggestions:
Red onion
Bell pepper
Cabbage
Carrots
Tenderstem broccoli
Beansprouts
2 chillies (1 red, 1 green)

To serve:
2 tbsp sesame seeds

Steps

- In a shallow bowl, combine all of the marinade ingredients and marinate the salmon for 1–2 hours, covered in the fridge.
- Preheat the oven to 190°C. Wrap the salmon in foil and put on a baking tray, flesh-side up, with the marinade, and cook in the oven for 15–20 minutes.
- In the last 5–10 minutes of the salmon cooking time, lightly fry the stir-fry vegetables in a wok with some sesame oil.
- Prepare the noodles by placing in a pan of hot water for 3–5 minutes over a low–medium heat, (or according to pack instructions) then drain and add to the wok.
- Squeeze lime juice into the wok with the vegetables and noodles, then plate up.
- Add the salmon on top of the vegetables and noodles and pour over any sauce left inside the foil.
- Sprinkle the sesame seeds on top.

Korma-style Curry

V, Veg, DF, GF

This recipe has been experimented with on numerous occasions. I wanted to recreate the sweet, warm and mildly spicy korma with a slight twist on the flavour.

SERVES 2

Ingredients
1 courgette
1 bell pepper

2 chicken breasts or 1 x 280g packet firm tofu
2 tbsp coconut oil
3 garlic cloves
2 large onions
1 x 400g tin coconut milk
Juice of ½ lime
2 tbsp coconut sugar
1 tbsp desiccated coconut
½–¼ tsp chilli powder or flakes (optional)
½ tsp ground cinnamon
1 tbsp ground almonds
½ tsp ground cardamom
150g brown rice
Sea salt and black pepper

For the spice mix:
1 heaped tsp ground ginger
2 tsp ground cumin
2 tsp ground coriander
1 tsp ground turmeric
1 heaped tsp mild curry powder

Serve with:
2 tbsp coconut yoghurt per person
Chopped fresh coriander leaves

Steps

- Place all the spice mix ingredients in a small bowl, then peel and chop the courgette and pepper.
- Slice the chicken breast and lightly fry in a pan until no longer pink (15–20 minutes) in 1 teaspoon of the coconut oil. Add

sea salt and black pepper and set aside in foil to keep warm. (Alternatively, you could bake in the oven on 200°C for 20 minutes.) If using tofu, cut into slices and lightly fry in a pan with 1 teaspoon of the coconut oil for 10–15 minutes, until golden and crispy, and set aside..

- Peel and chop the garlic cloves and onions, then cook in the same pan until golden (5–10 minutes) with the remaining oil. Add the cooked vegetables, then the spice mix, then add in the coconut milk and all the other ingredients apart from the rice, before adding the chicken. Stir and simmer for 30 minutes. (If using tofu, simply add it on top of the dish at the end).
- During this time, cook the brown rice, using the instructions on p. 88.
- Serve up with some coconut yoghurt and fresh coriander leaves.

Basil Emily Salad

V, Veg, DF, GF

This is perfect for a summer's day. It is full of healthy fats and a fresh, beachy Mediterranean taste. It is called 'Basil Emily' as I developed it in lockdown and home grew specific basil seeds named 'Basil Emily'.

SERVES 3

Ingredients

100g quinoa
2 garlic cloves
3 handfuls of kale, any kind

1 x 400g tin butter beans in water, drained and rinsed
10 cherry tomatoes
½ cucumber
8 sundried tomatoes
Handful of fresh basil
15–20g pine nuts
3 handfuls of spinach
1 avocado, peeled, stoned and chopped

Serve with:
Basil Salad Dressing (see p. 165)

Steps

- Preheat the oven to 190°C. Rinse the quinoa, put in a pan of salted boiling water and cook on a medium heat for 15–20 minutes or until tender. Drain, rinse and cool.
- While the quinoa is cooking, peel the garlic cloves and roast them whole in the oven for 10 minutes.
- Place some hot water in a pan and bring to the boil. Place the kale in a colander and steam on top of the boiling water for 3 minutes. The kale should be cooked, but not wilted. Rinse with cold water and place in a large mixing bowl.
- Add the butter beans to the bowl.
- Chop the cherry tomatoes, cucumber, sundried tomatoes, and fresh basil and place in the bowl. Mix well, then add the pine nuts and spinach.
- Add the quinoa to the mixing bowl once you have rinsed it with cold water and drained it. Stir everything together.
- Plate up the salad and add the chopped avocado on top. Then pour over the Basil Salad Dressing.

Kidney Bean Falafels

V, Veg, DF, GF

Delicious for lunchboxes and can be stored in the fridge for a few days.

SERVES 4 (MAKES 8)

Ingredients

80g quinoa, cooked and cooled (see method in the previous recipe, p. 134.)
1 x 400g tin kidney beans, cooked and rinsed
1 tbsp tomato purée
12 mint leaves
40g pumpkin seeds
½ tsp oregano
1 garlic clove, peeled and chopped
1 red onion, peeled and chopped
2 tbsp brown rice flour
1 tsp ground cumin
½ tsp ground coriander
¼ tsp cayenne pepper
Sea salt and black pepper

Steps

- Preheat your oven to 190°C.
- Blend all of the ingredients together in a food processor and mould into 8 patties.

- Place on a baking tray lined with baking parchment and bake for 15-20 minutes until golden brown, turning halfway through.
- Remove from the oven and serve with a salad, pitta breads, Tomato Relish Sauce (see p.163) and Cooling Mint Yoghurt Dip (see p. 162).

Victoria's Gut-healing Bone Broth

DF, GF

Autoimmunity nutritionist Victoria Jain shares her gut-healing recipe.

SERVES 4

Ingredients

250–500g bones from pasture-raised chicken or grass-fed beef (you can ask for these at your local butcher or use the carcass from a recent meal)
1 tsp olive oil
1.5 litres filtered or mineral water
2 tbsp apple cider vinegar (this helps to release nutrients from the bones)
2 carrots, chopped into cubes
2 celery sticks, chopped into cubes
1 white or red onion, finely diced
2 bay leaves
8 garlic cloves
½ bunch of parsley
4 tbsp fresh grated ginger
Sea salt and black pepper

Steps

- Heat a large pan or stockpot with the olive oil. Add the bones and lightly fry for 5 minutes.
- Add the water and vinegar to the pan and bring to the boil, then reduce the temperature, cover with the lid and leave to simmer very slowly for 8 hours, removing any white residue that builds using a large spoon.
- Add the remaining ingredients to the pan, apart from the fresh ginger, and simmer on a low heat for a further 2 hours.
- Remove the bones from the pan and strain the vegetables from the broth. Add the fresh grated ginger. (You could also opt to keep the vegetables as part of the broth, but use a soup blender for a smooth consistency.)
- ***Top tip:*** if you make a large batch of bone broth, you can transfer it to glass containers and freeze for a later date.

Harissa Lentil Pot

V, Veg, DF, GF

Deliciously spicy and warming dish that goes well with my Cooling Mint Yoghurt Dip (see p. 162).

SERVES 4

Ingredients

2 red onions
3 garlic cloves
5 carrots
1 bell pepper
1 courgette (optional)

150g mushrooms
Handful of cherry tomatoes
200g red split lentils
A drizzle of olive oil, for frying
2 tbsp tomato purée
2 x 400g tins chopped tomatoes
1 x 400g tin cannellini beans or chickpeas
3 tsp harissa spices
1 tsp ground cinnamon
½ tsp chilli flakes (optional)
½ tsp paprika
100g spinach
Sea salt and black pepper
Squeeze of lemon juice, to taste
Fresh coriander

Steps

- Peel, prepare and chop the vegetables.
- Rinse the lentils in cold water until the water runs clear. Fill a pan with the lentils and cold water. Bring to the boil and cook for 10 minutes, removing any foam, then cover and simmer for 5 minutes.
- Heat the oil in a large pan over a medium heat, fry the onions and garlic for 5–10 minutes and season with salt and pepper.
- Add the carrots, pepper, courgette (if using) mushrooms and cherry tomatoes in stages.
- During this time the lentils should have cooked. Rinse and add to the vegetables, along with the tomato purée, tinned tomatoes, cannellini beans and spices. Stir well.
- Stir in the spinach at the end.
- Serve with a squeeze of lemon juice, and garnish with fresh coriander.

Thai Green Curry

V, Veg, DF, GF

Aromatic and delicious flavours of a famous Thai dish.

SERVES 2

Ingredients

Choice of: cooked tofu, cod, prawns or chicken
2 bell peppers
2 tsp coconut oil
1 x 400g tin coconut milk
2 fresh lemongrass sticks (or, if not available, use 2 tsp dried)
2 kaffir lime leaves
1 pak choi, sliced
50g spinach

For the curry paste:

5 green chillies
3 garlic cloves
1 large piece of ginger (40g)
1 tsp ground cumin
5g fresh coriander or dried leaf
1 tbsp sesame oil
2 tsp tamari
½ tsp coriander seeds
Juice of ½ lime
Sea salt and black pepper

To serve:
Fresh coriander and cooked brown rice (see p. 79)

Steps

- Make the Thai green curry paste using a pestle-and-mortar setting on your food processor.
- Chop the peppers and your chosen main (tofu, cod, prawns or chicken).
- Fry the peppers for 5 minutes in coconut oil in a large pan over a medium heat.
- Add the curry paste and then your chosen main ingredient.
- Add in the coconut milk, lemongrass and kaffir lime leaves and stir well. Stir in the pak choi and spinach and simmer.
- Remove the lemongrass and kaffir lime leaves before serving.
- Serve with fresh coriander and cooked brown rice.

Slightly adjusted the steps to make time/a note for the cooked main ingredient:

Steps

- Make the Thai green curry paste using a pestle-and-mortar setting on your food processor. Cook your chosen main (tofu, cod, prawns or chicken), wrap to keep warm and place to one side.
- Chop the peppers and fry for 5 minutes in coconut oil in a large pan over a medium heat.
- Add the curry paste and then stir in your chosen main ingredient.
- Add in the coconut milk, lemongrass and kaffir lime leaves and stir well. Stir in the pak choi and spinach and simmer until wilted.
- Remove the lemongrass and kaffir lime leaves before serving.
- Serve with fresh coriander and cooked brown rice.

Desserts, Snacks and Treats

Sweet and Curry-spiced Mixed Nuts

V, Veg, DF, GF

I love snacks, and I'm always buying something snack-related . . . or inventing my own, such as these! This is an easy recipe to make a week's worth of sweet-and-spiced snacking nuts.

MAKES ABOUT 10 SERVINGS

Ingredients

500g packet of assorted nuts (cashews, almonds, walnuts, peanuts, pecans)
1 tbsp coconut oil
2 tbsp maple syrup
2 tbsp garam masala
½ tsp sea salt
½ tsp black pepper
½ tsp chilli powder or chilli flakes (to taste)

Steps

- Preheat the oven to 160°C. Place nuts in a large mixing bowl.
- Heat the coconut oil and maple syrup together in a saucepan on a medium heat until they form a liquid, then pour over the nuts, stirring in well.
- Add the garam masala, sea salt, pepper and chilli powder or flakes.

- Spread onto lined oven trays and cook for 25–30 minutes, turning over halfway through.
- Leave to cool and store in an airtight container. I often use old jars and take one to work with me each day of the week.

Cacao-dusted 'Truffles'

V, Veg, DF, GF

Oh, wow! These may not be truffles in the dairy-creamy sense, but they are just as addictive and have a dense yet soft centre.

MAKES 20

Ingredients

1 tbsp or 25ml melted coconut oil
12 Medjool dates (around 200g)
80g cashews
35g (or 1½ tbsp) date syrup
25g peanut butter
45g cacao powder
Sprinkle of sea salt

For the coating:
15g cacao powder
15g ground almonds
10g coconut sugar

Steps

- Blend all of the filling ingredients together in a food processor.
- Mould into 20 15–20g balls (Brussels-sprout-sized), and place on a plate.

- Mix all the coating ingredients together in a shallow dish.
- Roll each 'truffle' in the coating mixture.
- Leave in the fridge to set for 1 hour before serving.

Raspberry and Peanut Flapjacks

V, Veg, DF

You should have all the ingredients for these in the house already, ready to throw together. Makes for a good breakfast or a snack too. You can use any frozen berries.

MAKES 16 SMALL SQUARES OR 8 LARGER RECTANGLES

Ingredients

300g porridge oats
200g frozen raspberries
200ml almond milk (or any plant milk)
100g peanut butter
75g honey (or a vegan alternative – see p. 85), or more, if you prefer them sweeter

Steps

- Preheat the oven to 190°C.
- Combine all the ingredients in a bowl and stir well.
- Pour into a deep baking tray lined with baking parchment and flatten the top, then bake for 25–30 minutes, until it starts to look golden on top.
- Remove from the oven and leave to cool before cutting into 16 small squares or 8 rectangular pieces.

Raspberry Vegan 'Cheese' Cake

V, Veg, DF, GF

This recipe is a favourite of mine, and as long as you have a food processor, fridge and cake tin, you are good to go.

SERVES 8

Ingredients

For the base:

16 Deglet Nour dates (around 116g)
140g walnuts
30g flaxseeds
1 tsp French almond extract
2 tbsp maple syrup
1 level tbsp coconut oil, melted, plus extra for greasing
½ tsp ground cinnamon

For the cake:

225g raspberries
150g creamed coconut
4 tbsp maple syrup
100ml coconut milk from a carton
2 tbsp coconut oil

To finish:

Freeze-dried or fresh raspberries

Steps

- Grease a 20cm cake tin with coconut oil, or line with baking parchment.
- Blend all the ingredients for the base and press the mixture into the tin. Place in the freezer for 15 minutes.

- While the base is freezing, blend the cake layer ingredients together, then pour on top of the base. Freeze for 20 minutes.
- Top with fresh or freeze-dried raspberries and serve.

Bright Blueberry Muffins

Veg, DF, GF

Big blueberry muffins with a liquid gooey centre are my ultimate favourite choice at any coffee shop, but goodness knows how many additives are lurking in those – so I sought to recreate them myself at home.

MAKES 12

Ingredients

190g plain flour
150g unrefined natural caster sugar
2 tsp baking powder
¼ tsp sea salt
1 medium egg
80ml plant milk
90ml coconut oil, melted
1½ tsp vanilla essence
225g fresh blueberries
Coconut sugar, for sprinkling

Steps

- Preheat the oven to 200°C and line a cupcake tray with 12 paper cases.
- Whisk together the flour, sugar, baking powder and salt in a large bowl.

- In a Pyrex jug, mix together the wet ingredients, then combine the two mixtures before folding in the blueberries.
- Divide the mixture between the 12 cupcake cases – about 2–3 teaspoons in each.
- Sprinkle with coconut sugar, then bake for 15–20 minutes, turning partway through if the ones at the front are getting more cooked than those at the back.
- Remove from the oven when golden and serve.

Soft Banana Bread

Veg, DF, GF

I experimented with this recipe a lot during lockdown in 2020, as banana bread is such a comfort. The 'secret' ingredient here is the cardamom for a subtle sweet spice taste.

SERVES 8

Ingredients

Wet ingredients:

3 ripe bananas, mashed, plus 1 banana, sliced down the middle lengthways
2 eggs, whisked
2 tbsp coconut oil
1 tbsp honey (or a vegan alternative – see p. 85)
1 tbsp apple cider vinegar
1½ tbsp water

Dry ingredients:

1 tsp baking soda
1 tsp ground cinnamon

½ tsp ground nutmeg
¼ tsp ground cardamom
40g broken walnuts
150g buckwheat flour

Steps

- Preheat the oven to 180°C and brush a 500g loaf tin with dairy-free butter or coconut oil, or line with baking parchment.
- Combine all the wet ingredients apart from the sliced banana in a mixing bowl, then add the dry ingredients, folding in the buckwheat flour last.
- Pour the mixture into the loaf tin evenly, then place the sliced banana on top, with the inside facing up.
- Bake for 20–25 minutes, then remove from the oven and leave to rest before slicing.

Choco-avo-late Mousse

V, Veg, DF, GF

An alternative to creamy dairy mousse.

SERVES 4

Ingredients

2 avocados
5 heaped tsp cacao powder
250ml plant milk
1 tbsp coconut oil, melted
2–3 tsp maple syrup, depending on taste (add more if needed)
Pinch of sea salt

Toppings:
Coconut yoghurt
Walnuts
Strawberries
Manuka honey (or a vegan alternative – see p. 85)

Steps

- Blend all of the mousse ingredients and divide the mixture evenly between 4 glass dessert dishes. Place in the fridge.
- Add your choice of toppings before serving.

Vegan Mango Lassi

V, Veg, DF, GF

A refreshing drink with a cardamom kick.

SERVES 2

Ingredients

1 mango peeled, stone removed
Juice of ½ lime
200g coconut yoghurt
100ml plant milk
½–1 tsp ground cardamom powder
1–2 tsp maple syrup
Few ice cubes
1–2 tbsp chia or flaxseeds (optional)

Steps

- Blend all of the ingredients together.

Baked and Spiced Chickpeas

V, Veg, DF, GF

A crispy, savoury and moreish snack.

SERVES 4

Ingredients

1 x 400g tin chickpeas
1 tbsp olive oil
2 tsp smoked paprika
2 tsp garlic granules
1 tsp ground cumin
½ tsp oregano
½ tsp cayenne pepper
Sea salt and black pepper

Steps

- Preheat the oven to 180°C.
- Drain and rinse the chickpeas and place in a bowl.
- Stir in the olive oil and spices.
- Spread the chickpeas evenly over a lined baking tray.
- Roast for 40 minutes until crispy, and leave to cool before eating.

Fudgy Sweet-potato Brownies

V, Veg, DF, GF

Super-squidgy and delicious brownies.

MAKES 16 SQUARES

Ingredients

2 large sweet potatoes (around 380g)
3 heaped tbsp cacao powder
150g nut butter
8 tbsp maple syrup
100g dates, chopped
150ml coconut oil, melted
90g brown rice flour
½ tsp baking powder
125g broken walnuts
300ml plant milk
Sprinkle of sea salt

Steps

- Preheat the oven to 190°C and line a deep baking tray with baking parchment or grease with melted coconut oil.
- Peel and chop the sweet potatoes into the smallest chunks you can manage, then boil in a pan of water for 10 minutes, until soft enough for a fork to go through the pieces.
- Drain the sweet potato well, mash in a large mixing bowl and stir in all the remaining ingredients.
- Pour the mixture into the prepared tin and bake for 25–30 minutes, turning the tray around halfway through the cooking

time. They should be soft and squidgy, but not liquidy inside. Allow to cool before cutting into 16 squares.

- Serve as they are, or with a spoonful of coconut yoghurt.

Deconstructed Pear Crumble

V, Veg, DF, GF

Sounds simple and it is – *really* easy and *really* tasty! You could also use rhubarb when it is in season; my sister grows it in her garden.

SERVES 2

Ingredients

1 tsp ground cinnamon
Pinch of ground nutmeg
1 tsp honey (or a vegan alternative – see p. 85)
1 tsp coconut sugar
½ tsp oil (coconut, melted or olive)
2 conference pears, peeled and halved

For the toppings:
Homemade granola
2 tbsp mix of walnuts and pecans
Coconut yoghurt
Maple syrup

Steps

- Preheat the oven to 180°C.
- Cut a large piece of foil and sprinkle the spices, honey and coconut sugar on it, with a drizzle of oil.

- Rub the pear halves in the mixture, then wrap them up in the foil, and bake for 25–30 minutes.
- Serve with your choice of toppings. You can also store in the fridge for the next day and eat cold.

Dad's Essential-mineral-fuelled Snack

V, Veg, DF, GF

My dad used to keep a Tupperware in his glove box, jam-packed with Brazil nuts and raisins. Brazil nuts contain a significant amount of selenium and they are also packed full of zinc.

SERVES 1

Ingredients

28g (about 10) Brazil nuts
30g raisins

Steps

- Pour both ingredients into a chosen container (plastic-free or reusable if you can).
- Eat. Together. It might sound a little strange at first, but place both a Brazil nut and a raisin in your mouth at the same time. Honestly, you won't be able to eat one without the other ever again.

Drinks, Juices and Smoothies

All the recipes in this section are: V (or can be made V), Veg, DF, GF

Matcha Moment

Making time for a matcha moment has become part of my self-care routine during the week – whether it is with a hot or cold latte or in a smoothie, it's both rejuvenating and nutritious (see p. 33).

SERVES 1

Ingredients

½–1 tsp matcha green tea powder, plus extra for sprinkling
2–3 tbsp warm water
200ml water or plant milk, hot or cold
½ tsp honey (or a vegan alternative – see p. 85) – if you are trying it for the first time it may seem quite bitter

> Traditional Japanese tea-ceremony utensils (optional, but worth investing if you enjoy it!):
> *Chawan:* small tea bowl; alternative: large, wide tea mug or small bowl
> *Chashaku:* bent bamboo spoon; alternative: teaspoon
> *Chasen:* special bamboo whisk; alternative: small baking whisk

Steps

- To prepare your matcha in the traditional Japanese way, measure the matcha tea powder into your *chawan* with a *chashaku*. You could use a small sieve at this point to get rid of any large lumps.
- Add the 2–3 tablespoons of warm water and gently whisk using a *chasen* from left to right, to form a smooth and silky consistency, removing any clumping.
- Heat the 200ml water or plant milk in a frother machine or in a small saucepan, no higher than 70°C. (Skip this part if you're having a cold matcha.)
- Add the cold or hot liquid to the *chawan*.
- Add the honey to taste if you like it, then a few sprinkles of matcha green tea powder on the top for decoration, or ice if it is cold.

Nausea-knocking Peppermint Tea

Feeling nauseous? Unsettled tummy? Peppermint tea has anti-spasmodic properties that can treat the feelings of nausea and prevent vomiting. May help if you're on methotrexate tablets.

SERVES 2

Ingredients

Handful of fresh mint leaves

600ml hot water

Honey (or a vegan alternative – see p. 85), to taste

Steps

- Place the mint leaves and hot water in a teapot with a strainer inside.
- Let the mint leaves steep for 5–10 minutes before pouring. Add a teaspoon of organic honey to sweeten if needed.

Chocolate M*lk Shake

Vegan and plant-based chocolatey milkshake, for a treat alternative.

SERVES 1

Ingredients

1 banana
200ml plant milk
50ml water
1 heaped tsp cacao powder
¼ tsp ground cinnamon
1 tbsp nut butter
2 tsp honey (or a vegan alternative – see p. 85)
2 Medjool dates (optional)

Steps

- Blend all the ingredients together. Chill or drink immediately.

Ginger Kick (Banana, Mango, Ginger)

A vibrant drink to kick off the day, or to have as a booster later on in the day.

SERVES 2

Ingredients
2 bananas
½ fresh mango, peeled, or a handful of frozen chunks
1 tsp ground ginger
2 tbsp honey (or a vegan alternative – see p. 85)
300ml plant milk
150ml water

Steps
- Blend all of the ingredients together. Refrigerate and then drink!

Strawberries and 'Cream'

This actually tastes like strawberries and cream – what a treat!

SERVES 2

Ingredients
50g cashews
1 banana
235g strawberries
2 Medjool dates
3 tbsp coconut yoghurt
250ml plant milk
1 tsp honey or maple syrup

Steps

- Soak the cashews in boiling water for 5 minutes, then drain and rinse in cold water.
- Blend the cashews with the rest of the ingredients. Drink immediately or when desired.

Pecan Pie Shake

Pecan pie in a drink.

SERVES 1

Ingredients

1 banana
½ tsp maca powder
1–2 Medjool dates
¼ tsp vanilla extract
1–2 tbsp nut butter
3 large dollops coconut yoghurt (or 200ml plant milk if you don't have coconut yoghurt)
25ml water
7 pecans, plus extra to serve
½ tsp honey (or a vegan alternative – see p. 85)
2 tbsp oats
Pinch of ground cinnamon

Steps

- Blend all the ingredients together, then top with extra pecans too. Drink immediately.

Mango and Raspberry Refresher

If you can get ripe mangoes when they're in season – June, July – it's worth it!

SERVES 2

Ingredients
2 mangoes, peeled and stoned
70g fresh or frozen raspberries
1 tsp lime juice
150ml coconut plant milk

Steps

- Blend all the ingredients together. Drink immediately or when desired!

Maca Smoothie

For a quick reminder of the many powers of maca powder, see p. 74.

SERVES 2

Ingredients
1 heaped tsp maca
1 heaped tsp raw cacao powder
2 bananas
1–2 handfuls frozen or fresh mango
250ml plant milk

Steps

- Blend all the ingredients together. Drink immediately and enjoy!

Indulgent Hot Cacao

Cacao and not cocoa – see p. 74!

SERVES 1

Ingredients

1 tbsp cacao powder
1 tbsp maple syrup
¼ tsp vanilla extract
Pinch of ground cinnamon
200ml plant milk
Pinch of sea salt

Steps

- Combine all the ingredients together in a pan over a medium heat. Whisk gently and stir until smooth and piping hot, around 3–5 minutes, then pour into a mug and serve. Drink immediately and enjoy!

Berry Power

Berries mixed for a super-berry boost here, as a morning or afternoon snack.

SERVES 1

Ingredients
60g blueberries
60g raspberries
60g blackberries
60g strawberries
1 banana
1 tsp honey (or a vegan alternative – see p. 85)
150ml plant milk

Steps

- Blend all the ingredients together and enjoy immediately.

Warming Chai

Plenty of warming anti-inflammatory spices are combined in this autumnal drink.

SERVES 2

Ingredients
350ml plant milk
150ml water

2 cinnamon sticks
2 star anise
1 whole nutmeg (or ½ tsp ground)
2 cardamom pods
Pinch of black peppercorns
15g freshly grated or finely sliced ginger
½ tsp ground allspice
½ tsp vanilla essence
Black tea leaves (optional)
1 tbsp honey (or a vegan alternative – see p. 85)

Steps

- Heat the plant milk and water with all of the spices over a low–medium heat and gradually bring to the boil (this takes 4–5 minutes). Lower the heat and simmer gently for another 4–5 minutes.
- Add the black tea, if using, and brew on a low heat for 2–3 minutes.
- Add the honey, then carefully strain into a jug, before dividing the liquid between 2 mugs. Add to a milk frother, if you'd like it frothy!

Sauces, Sides and Dips

All the recipes in this section are: V (or can be made V), Veg, DF, GF

Cooling Mint Yoghurt Dip

This minty dip goes especially well with the recipes on pp. 135 and 137.

SERVES 2

Ingredients
100g coconut yoghurt
¼ cucumber, grated
Handful of fresh mint, chopped (or 2 tsp dried)
Sea salt and black pepper

Steps
- Fill a 250ml glass jar a third of the way with coconut yoghurt, then add the cucumber, mint, sea salt and black pepper and stir well.

Butter-bean Burger Sauce

This is a creamy alternative to mayonnaise.

MAKES 4 SERVINGS

Ingredients
1 x 400g tin butter beans, drained and rinsed
1 tbsp coconut oil, melted

100ml plant milk
1 tsp honey (or a vegan alternative – see p. 85)
1 tbsp tamari
1 tsp garlic paste
Small handful of fresh coriander

Steps

- Blend all the ingredients together. (You may want more or less plant milk, depending on preferred thickness.)

Tomato Relish Sauce

Goes really well with the Cajun Salmon or Chickpea Burgers on pp. 123–6 and pp. 126–7).

MAKES 2 SERVINGS

Ingredients
1 large round tomato
3 tbsp tomato purée
3 tbsp water
1 tsp balsamic vinegar
Pinch of ground cumin
2 tsp olive oil
1 tsp fresh chopped coriander
¼ tsp chilli flakes
½ tsp honey (or a vegan alternative – see p. 85)
½ tsp garlic granules
Sea salt and black pepper

Steps

- Chop the tomato and place in a small bowl with the rest of the ingredients. Stir well. Store covered, in a small bowl or jar in the fridge for up to 3 days.

Homemade Coleslaw

A delicious side dish to go with burgers, fritters, salads and all sorts.

SERVES 6

Ingredients

5 carrots (around 350g)
½ white cabbage (around 475g)
2 tsp wholegrain mustard
200ml mayonnaise or coconut yoghurt
2 tsp coconut sugar
2 tbsp apple cider vinegar
Sea salt and black pepper

Steps

- Peel and grate the carrots. If you have a food processor, use the grater setting to do this for ease.
- Destalk and chop the white cabbage into strips, chunky and thin.
- Place the carrots and cabbage in a bowl along with the rest of the coleslaw ingredients and stir well until fully combined.

Basil Salad Dressing

Use this to dress any salad. It goes especially well with the Basil Emily Salad recipe on p. 133.

MAKES 4 SERVINGS

Ingredients
135ml extra virgin olive oil
½ tbsp apple cider vinegar
½ tsp garlic granules (or 1 garlic clove, roasted and chopped)
10g fresh basil, chopped
1 tsp balsamic vinegar
½ tsp dried oregano
½ tsp lime juice
½ tsp sea salt
½ tsp black pepper

Steps

- Mix all of the ingredients in a jug and whisk well.

Hummus

Serve with peppers, celery, cucumber, carrots or warm sourdough slices.

MAKES 3 DIPPING BOWLS

Ingredients
2 garlic cloves
2 x 400g tins chickpeas, drained
1 tsp ground cumin
2 tbsp tahini

100ml water
100ml olive oil
Sea salt and black pepper

Steps

- Roast the garlic cloves for 10 minutes, skin on, at 200°C, then peel.
- Mix all the ingredients for the hummus in a food processor. Store covered in the fridge.

Tahini Salad Dressing

Sweet, salty, with a sesame nutty flavour. Great with roasted vegetables and salads like the Rainbow Buddha Bowl on pp. 108–9.

MAKES 4 SERVINGS

Ingredients
2 tbsp tahini
6 tbsp olive oil
½ tsp garlic granules
½ tsp ground cumin
1 tbsp balsamic vinegar
2 tsp honey (or a vegan alternative – see p. 96)
1 tbsp apple cider vinegar
½ tsp chilli flakes (optional)
Sea salt and black pepper
2 tbsp water

Steps

- Place all the ingredients in a lidded jar and shake. Use immediately or cover and store in the fridge for up to 5 days.

6

Pain Management

'Pain is inevitable. Suffering is optional.'

Haruki Murakami, author

All of us, arthritics or not, have endured the distressing and uncomfortable feeling of pain at one time or another, however it manifests: from cuts (like cutting your hand open while destoning an avocado!), burns and bruises, headaches and joint afflictions, dull or sharp, burning or stabbing, tingling or aching, acute or chronic . . .

Even though it can vary from person to person, and even within the same person at different times, there is a unifying theory of pain: it all originates with inflammation and the body's inflammatory response, and those pro-inflammatory cytokines we met in Chapter 1 are involved in the process.

Like most of us, when you are in agony all you can think about is how to kick pain out of the door rather than invite it in for a cup of tea and spend time getting to know it. But the more you can understand about pain, the better equipped you will be to deal with it (using the tips in this chapter).

Acute vs Chronic Pain: What's the Difference?

Acute pain usually exits shortly after it arrives – say, when you accidentally touch a hot stove or stub your toe. Chronic pain, on the other hand – well, it settles in and stays the night. In the case of chronic-pain syndromes, such as arthritis, the pain is accompanied by chronic inflammation as well.

Managing both pain and inflammation is the red thread throughout this book. Living with chronic pain is like walking (or crawling) uphill. On some days, you may be able to really push on, while on others you might need to stop and rest. Then, the following day, you may be on top of it before, a few days later, bumping and rolling back down. It's a cycle. It's up. It's down. It's unpredictable. And partnered with its unpredictable nature is the strength of the pain – a relief when it is bearable and fades into the edges of your day, but sucking up your energy when it's overwhelming and takes up space.

A tree of pain

On high-pain days it's like a whole tree has taken root and it is all you are able to feel or think about. On medium-pain days you may only notice a branch or two, while on low-pain days perhaps only the presence of the tree's leaves.

If there is a low-pain day, you will likely choose to make the most of the day – perhaps, you'll venture out into the fresh air and embark on a walk or spend an evening out with friends. On a high-pain day, you can find me indoors with my feet up, diverting my mind by listening to, reading or watching something, and soothing my pain with some of the remedies listed in this chapter. My intention here is not to undermine the advice or treatment given to you by your doctor; but in more cases than not, it is beneficial to find your own way of managing your arthritis and to feel as though you have a handle on your pain – and my wish is that you will feel the need to pop painkiller pills less frequently as a result.

Consider this chapter as tea-time with your old friend pain. It is time to learn all about how it manifests and behaves within your body. Turns out, more people have this unwanted guest than you may realise, with around a third of adults in England reporting chronic pain due to musculoskeletal conditions such as arthritis. In most cases, chronic pain also instigates other symptoms like depression, which we will unpick further in Chapter 9. The economic burden of chronic pain is huge, yet the medical approach for pain management has been slow to progress.

The 'bio-psycho-social' tripod

In 1977, American doctor and psychiatrist George Engel shifted our understanding of pain into a more holistic 'bio-psycho-social model', altering the medical approach to pain for the better. Previously, pain was only dealt with at a biological level disregarding the social and psychological drivers. If you imagine pain as a tripod, it cannot stand up without all three legs, can it? Well, the same could be said for the bio-psycho-social model: pain has to be seen as an experience that results from all three 'legs': biology (DNA make-up), psychology (personality, emotions, behaviour) and sociology (culture, experiences, family, socioeconomics).

So it is no wonder, then, that we all feel pain differently. Traumatic childhood experiences, post-traumatic stress disorder (PTSD) and stress have all been strongly connected as either contributing factors to the onset of RA, or aggravating its symptoms. Could losing my dad at a young age be one of the contributing factors to the onset of my arthritis? It is hard to know for sure, but what I can tell you is that when I am stressed, upset or feeling low, my pain and symptoms are always worse than usual.

A Conversation About Pain

Steve Haines, author of *Pain Is Really Strange*, has been working as a bodyworker for over 20 years, is a registered chiropractor and teaches trauma-releasing exercises (TRE) and cranial work globally. Understanding the science of pain and trauma has transformed his approach to healing, and I spoke to him about it:

Q. How does pain work?

A. Pain is strange, in that it is non-linear and quickly becomes amplified over and above what is happening in the tissues. There is a modern definition of pain that hinges on safety:

- Pain is an alarm system, a warning signal, emerging when your brain decides that something is unsafe or wrong:
    - a stressful situation
    - trauma
    - an injury.
- When the brain is screaming 'danger, danger' in a 'fight-or-flight' mode, as a survival reflex it diverts things away from:
    - growth and repair
    - and long-term projects in the body.

- The pain will be associated with an amplified stress response:
  - o increased heart rate
  - o altered digestive system
  - o a pause on normal functions – our resources are diverted while in this state; it is conscious and semi-conscious, led by the central nervous system.
- Short-term acute pain protects us from danger.
- Long-term chronic pain has no discernible purpose.
  - o With chronic pain, the alarm system becomes too sensitive and the brain's response becomes automatic, irrespective of what messages are actually being sent to it. So, your pain may not always be indicative of what is actually going on in your body, having become an unconscious habit whereby the body is overprotecting itself.

Q. What about for inflammatory conditions?

A. In the last 10 to 15 years, we have learned that the immune system also has protective reflexes. If there is a perception of threat inside your body (the alarm system), not only do we have conscious pain experience and the stress response, as described above, but also, gearing up to protect us is the inflammatory response.

Led by the immune system, inflammation is typically a protective reflex (see Chapter 3). But like persistent pain, the inflammation may continue to run even though the danger has passed. Steve offers that many AIDs or inflammatory conditions are rooted in this overprotective inflammatory reflex that was once useful, but then becomes a habitual and unconscious experience, continuing in the background even if the physical affliction has subsided.

Inflammation is a powerful response, but when it is poorly controlled and spreads to other areas of the body, then it becomes a problem. And this is how we may think of inflammatory conditions that are associated with chronic pain: we have got an out-of-control, habitual inflammatory response, but if we can safely de-stress the body, we can begin to regain control.

The vagus nerve, the longest nerve in the body (running from the brain to the abdomen), plays a significant part, and here's why . . . It oversees a vast array of crucial bodily functions, including control of mood, immune response, digestion and heart rate. It carries an extensive range of signals and information from the digestive system and organs to the brain, and vice versa. It has an important role in the relationship between the gut, the brain and inflammation. Vagus-nerve stimulation (VNS) and meditation techniques have shown to be beneficial in mood and anxiety disorders, and for conditions associated with increased inflammation, such as RA, representing an important link between nutrition and inflammatory diseases.

Steve further notes that the vagus nerve is one of the primary regulators of inflammatory conditions and is most efficient when we are prosocial, engaged with others, feeling safe and connected to our bodies and have the capacity to sleep and rest. Hence, when we are stressed or sleep-deprived, our inflammation, pain and symptoms may be exacerbated.

Q. What about arthritic pain in particular?

A. Advances in preclinical research have led to significant progress in understanding the processes underlying the development of arthritis pain. As Steve says, the pain hypersensitivity may persist after the inflammation has ended, and consequently this manifests as dysfunctional pathological changes in the central nervous system. The alarm has not turned off and adjusted appropriately to the situation, leading to chronic pain.

Q. What can I do about it?

A. Now that you understand more about the processing of pain, reducing the stress and inflammatory response and ensuring a happy gut are imperative. So, next up is a look at complementary and alternative medicine (CAM) approaches for arthritis pain, categorised as follows:

- Herbs and minerals: oral and topical treatments
- At-home therapies
- Out-of-home therapies
- Tips from Steve

Herbs and Minerals: Oral and Topical Treatments

An array of natural elements, in the form of herbs and minerals, have been used in easing arthritic pain and symptoms. The following is a breakdown of some of these.

Epsom salt

Magnesium sulphate, or Epsom salt, is not to be used in cooking, as it's not really a 'salt' at all, being made up of magnesium, sulphur and oxygen. Magnesium is essential for relieving stress and inducing a good night's sleep, plus it is both medicative and therapeutic in alleviating pain, swelling and sore muscles. I love taking an Epsom-salt bath to relieve my arthritic pain.

The theory is that the Epsom salts treat the body from the outside in, and the magnesium is absorbed by passing through the skin. Immersion in a bath filled with Epsom salt is alleged to supplement magnesium levels, although this is not scientifically proven. If you want to check out the benefits for yourself, look for high-quality pharmaceutical-grade salts sourced from reserves that are around 800 million years old. An Epsom-salt bath should be done in the evening, right before bed, two or more times a week. This is how you do it:

- Dissolve 2–3 mugs of high-quality Epsom salt in a bath of hot water – as hot as you can bear. (**Note**: if you have any pre-existing heart or blood-pressure condition, you should not bathe in very hot water.)
- Do not add any bath products to the water.
- Get in the bath, lie still and relax. Or, if you feel you are able to, you can exercise your body lightly from joint to joint, using some of the range-of-motion exercises on p. 205. It should be easier to do them in the heat and weightlessness of the water.
- Stay as long as you can, if you have the time; otherwise, 20 minutes should be sufficient.
- You could also try some of the breathing and meditation methods in Chapter 9, listen to relaxing music, light candles and even soak up an episode of your favourite podcast while you soak too.

- Dry yourself quickly and get into bed to keep warm. It should make you feel relaxed and tired. It is an ideal way to unwind, a wonderful pain relief and an aid to a good night's sleep.

If you don't have time for a bath, use the sink or a deep bowl and fill it with hot water and a cup of Epsom salt. Dip your affected areas in (hands, feet, ankles) for 10–15 minutes to soothe and relieve any pain. Dry gently and moisturise afterwards.

Cannabidiol (CBD)

Globally, cannabis has been used for medical purposes as far back as 2900 BC, treating joint pain, muscle spasms and gout – to name a few. Cannabis-based medicines (when prescribed by a registered specialist doctor) have been legalised in a number of countries.

However, CBD does not equal cannabis (I'm not trying to get any of you in trouble). CBD oil is extracted from the flowers and leaves of the cannabis or hemp plant, rather than the plant as a whole. CBD is one of the fastest-growing industries in the realm of health and wellness, showing huge promise in the alleviation of chronic pain, skin conditions such as psoriasis and sleep disturbance.

The whole plant contains all kinds of compounds and more than 120 natural phytochemicals, cannabinoids, have been identified – each with its own benefits. The two main ones are THC and CBD.

- **THC:** creates the famous sensation of getting 'high' and is the main psychoactive cannabinoid found in cannabis. THC assists with chronic-pain symptoms and may enhance the effects of CBD, but if the THC content is more than 0.2 per cent, it would require a prescription.

- **CBD:** is considered non-psychoactive, and CBD products can be taken without a prescription.

Where can I buy CBD?

CBD is available as oral drops, topical creams, transdermal patches, vapourisers, balms and teas. I love CBD tea and find it very calming; I have oral drops for pain relief and a balm to soothe too. Both oral and topical application of CBD have shown therapeutic potential for the relief of arthritic symptoms and inflammation in preliminary studies. When it comes to buying it, CBD will usually be listed as 'cannabidiol', 'full-spectrum hemp', 'hemp' oil or paste. Although there is a need for larger, well-controlled clinical trials for the treatment of musculoskeletal pain/systemic autoimmune diseases, there is potential.

Peppermint

Peppermint leaves have been used across the world for several thousand years to relieve stress-related symptoms, pain and nausea (the latter often being a side effect of arthritis medication, such as DMARDs).

Peppermint has a high menthol content (40 per cent) that activates the cold-sensitive receptors in our skin, nose and mouth, creating a cooling sensation. A delicious way to enjoy the polyphenol health benefits of mint is by drinking a fresh mint tea (see p. 154), which I find to be really calming when taking medication. Alternatively, it may soothe your swollen joints in the form of peppermint oil balms, creams and sprays. An inexpensive and effective menthol-based product is biofreeze, or Tiger Balm.

Aloe vera

For millennia, cultures all over the world have used aloe vera for medicinal purposes. Queen Cleopatra even used it as part of her regular beauty regime. Used to aid wounds or soothe skin, for example (like the lobster-red sunburn I endure seasonally), it's anti-inflammatory (producing effects similar to NSAIDs), anti-arthritic, anti-rheumatoid and antioxidant. Aloe vera has been used traditionally as an arthritis treatment (in topical and oral form) for centuries, providing pain relief when applied directly to swollen, inflamed and painful joints.

Gels, creams, sprays, lotions and drinks can all be derived from the plant's fleshy leaves. What's more, aloe vera is highly nutritious. Grow it at home or buy it fresh if you can. The gooey and sticky gel can be added to smoothies or salsa and the skin can be sliced and added to a summer salad. **Note**: be sure to remove the thin layer of yellow liquid between the skin and the gel of the leaf, as it can have serious side effects if overconsumed.

Capsaicin

Peppers are pretty popular, consumed all over the world as additions to curries, salads and stir-fries. But besides their culinary uses, peppers are also valued for their nutraceutical and medicinal purposes. Capsaicin is one of the active phytochemicals in the pepper family with antioxidant, anti-inflammatory and antimicrobial activities.

Capsaicin cream or gel, to be applied topically – on to the skin of the affected joint – is a natural pain-relief therapy, recommended for arthritics by the WHO. GPs may prescribe it to OA patients in particular, as it has been found to be an effective therapy for OA pain in four separate trials. Used in this form, the capsaicin is four times more effective than a placebo gel in decreasing OA pain and tenderness. Capsaicin is thought to reduce pain through blocking the transmission of pain signals and the activation of inflammatory cytokines in joints. For best results, applying a pea-size amount of capsaicin cream to your affected joints up to four times a day is recommended, and no more than every four hours during the day.

Glucosamine

Naturally found in our cartilage, glucosamine is a popular dietary and topical treatment for alleviating OA. Glucosamine provides natural building blocks for growth, repair and maintenance of cartilage, and our ability to produce it may become impaired with age. Some assert that glucosamine reduces the deterioration of cartilage, relieves pain and improves joint mobility. Glucosamine can be found in topical creams and gels, or in oral capsules, at your local health-food store or online.

At-home Therapies

Many of the herbs and minerals, topical and oral remedies described above can be accessed away from home, on the go – perhaps you can carry them in your pocket or purse for when you need them the most. The following remedies may be a little more difficult to do away from home.

Heat/cold therapy

Heat (say, a hot bath) or cold (ice wraps, for example) can feel good when we are hurting, *but why?*

In our bodies, TRP (transient receptor potential) channels are thought to behave like microscopic thermometers, and pain researchers hold that activating certain of these may create similar effects to applying ice or heat packs to an injured joint in terms of reducing pain sensation.

- **Cold:** some TRP channels are activated by cool temperatures and or things that create sensations of coolness, like menthol (peppermint).
- **Hot:** some TRP channels are triggered by heat, or by compounds like capsaicin (peppers), piperine (black pepper) and garlic (allicin) or even cannabinoids (see p. 175).

I have gel packs that can be stored in the freezer or heated in the microwave. Pharmacist Raj Vara adds that heat relaxes the muscles and connective tissues, promoting blood flow and healing.

For extreme-temperature therapies, you could try infrared light therapy (for the scorching hot) or cryotherapy (for the freezing cold) – but be sure to speak to your doctor before doing so.

Compression

Compression therapy in the form of gloves, elbow or knee supports is widely recommended or prescribed by rheumatologists for those living with various forms of arthritis. Compression clothing is worn to improve blood flow, as well as to lessen any pain or swelling, or to function as a brace, enabling more control and comfort when walking, for instance. Compression designs comprise two main features: applying pressure (pressure therapy) and providing warmth (heat therapy).

Efficiency and comfort are paramount, so speak to your doctor before trying or using compression-therapy products. It is also recommended to take them off at night for sleeping.

Transcutaneous electrical nerve stimulation (TENS)

Safe, drug-free and pain reducing, transcutaneous electrical nerve stimulation (TENS) machines operate by sending small electrical currents to particularly painful areas of the body through sticky electrode pads placed on the surface of the skin.

The electrical currents are low voltage, but range in strength, frequency and length. I found that my right ankle, where I feel more pain, required a higher voltage and frequency than my left, for instance.

The electric impulses are said to halt and numb pain. There are various theories as to why this works: by 'rubbing' the pain away, blocking our perception of pain or simply by distraction. But speaking from experience, the TENS machine seems to do all of the above – my pain feels relieved when using it, both by the sensation of it and the distraction it provides, and I can feel the effects of it afterwards too.

TENS therapy has been used or is being studied to relieve both chronic and acute pain and is recommended as a short-term pain relief for RA and OA, with benefits demonstrated for both in small clinical trials. Pooled results from 32 studies analysing TENS for chronic musculoskeletal pain disorders, such as RA, OA or AS, indicated a significant decrease in pain compared with a placebo.

A TENS can be used for 15–20 minutes at a time, several times per day; however, some find that using them for hours at a time with breaks in between is more suitable for them. Remedies like this will not work for everyone, so speak to your doctor first to ensure it is the right approach to managing your pain safely.

Out-of-home Therapies

Out-of-home therapies are any treatments that require someone or something else to do the treatment for you. These vary in their ability to provide relief, and what works for your pain might not even touch the edges for someone else. Or you might receive treatment from an inexperienced massage therapist before finding that intuitive magician with melting hand moves.

If you have the time and the disposable income to try some of these therapies (or if your GP can see the necessity for them in your treatment plan), here is a breakdown of the key ones I have come across for our condition, but this list is not exhaustive.

Acupuncture

Acupuncture is a regularly prescribed medical treatment, carried out by a trained professional such as a physiotherapist or an acupuncturist. When I first heard of this 3,000-year-old Chinese-medicine therapy, I naively (or rightly) considered it a little strange to willingly allow someone to insert needles into your skin for long periods of time. It sounded positively *awful* – how could doing this feel good? Wouldn't it hurt or sting? And could the needles get stuck? These and similar thoughts flooded my head before I had my first session. Turns out, it is not the intimidating painful procedure I was picturing, and it felt peculiarly relaxing.

So, what exactly are these acupuncture needles and what do they do? Well, they are solid, metallic and flexible, as fine as a strand of hair. And the technique involves gently penetrating the skin with the needles at specific points on the body, depending on the target area, inserting them to a point that produces a sensation of pressure, or an ache. Acupuncture points are considered to stimulate the central nervous system, releasing the body's natural painkillers into the muscles, spinal cord and brain, as well as encouraging healing and boosting overall wellbeing. Although the method of acupuncture is not always based on hard scientific evidence, studies suggest it may help to ease chronic pain or reduce and prevent the frequency of headaches.

Massage

Massage may still have connotations of a luxurious day at the spa – candlelight and incense, the soft, gentle voice of the massage therapist and a fluffy towel-cum-bathrobe – but having now become more mainstream it may be less spa-like and more like a visit to the GP or physiotherapist. Sure, it can be relaxing, but it can also feel uncomfortable, sore or tense – albeit a good kind of discomfort. (Depending on the type of massage treatment you choose or need the most, it can either be a treat or a bit of an endurance test, making you feel good *and* like jelly afterwards.) A therapeutic treatment lasting from half an hour to an hour, its purpose varies from pain relief to sport recovery, or simply relaxation.

Each form of massage has its own benefits, but typically, a massage therapist will use physical, hands-on movements such as pressing, kneading or stretching tissues on target areas of the body. Using differing pressures and techniques, the intention is to manipulate the soft tissues and muscles, releasing any tension, aches or soreness. Practised for at least 4,000 years, massage therapy considers the body holistically and is designed to encourage healing and provide relief from injury, stress, pain and other acute and chronic conditions. According to the *Encyclopedia of Stress*, it may be able to reduce anxiety, tension, stress and depression, alongside increasing circulation and inducing a sense of overall wellbeing.

While large and rigorous investigations are needed into the effectiveness of massage therapy as a remedy for people living with arthritis, so far it has been shown to provide relief in people with OA, RA and AS. The following are some of the key types of massage, all of which should be delivered by qualified massage therapists.

- **Swedish massage** Perhaps the most widely known 'traditional' form, the Swedish massage is designed to soothe muscles, improve circulation and encourage relaxation with gentle, light massage strokes, primarily working on the surface level of the body, using massage oil.

Variations of the Swedish massage:

- **Hot-stone massage** Smooth, flat, heated stones are placed on specific parts of your body, depending on the focus of the treatment, either replacing or in addition to hand techniques. It may improve sleep quality and reduce sleep disturbance.
- **Aromatherapy massage** 'Essential oils' from herb, tree and flower extracts are diluted into the massage oil or lotion used. Absorbed through your skin or inhaled through a diffuser, the scent and properties of the essential oils have a range of purposes, alleged to ease anxiety, aid sleep and reduce inflammation and pain. Essential oils are extremely concentrated, so they should always be diluted in a carrier oil or water. If you have allergies or sensitivities, speak to your doctor ahead of any treatment. There are more than 90 types, but here are some of my 'anti-arthritic' favourites:
  - Eucalyptus
  - Lavender
  - Bergamot
  - Ylang ylang
  - Patchouli
  - Rosemary
  - Chamomile
  - Frankincense
  - Peppermint
  - Ginger

- **Deep-tissue massage** This form of massage focuses on the deeper layers of your muscles, from tension to 'knots' and muscular and joint pain. You should feel an equal balance of discomfort and soothing pressure. Primarily used to treat both chronic and acute pain (such as sports injuries), it uses massage oil and may include the use of elbows or forearms, in combination with the hands. After one of these sessions, I feel as though I have been spun and dropped out of a tumble dryer – a little shaken up, but soft and warm, like a chocolate you've left in your pocket for too long.
- **Shiatsu massage** 'Shiatsu' is derived from the Japanese term for 'finger pressure'. In this therapy, finger pressure is applied to the acupressure points on the body (the same ones used in acupuncture), moving from one point to another in a rhythmic sequence. No massage oil is required, so loose and comfortable clothing is usually worn throughout.

Physical therapies

The world of mainstream and complementary physical therapies can be a little puzzling. My grandma sang the praises of her chiropractor, and I said, 'But, I've seen an osteopath before and a physiotherapist. How is a chiropractor any different?' Needless to say, neither of us at the time was 100 per cent sure how to distinguish between them, as all three are qualified to attend to musculoskeletal pain. But here's the difference:

- **Chiropractor**: mainly focuses on the alignment of the spine and central nervous system

- **Osteopath**: centres around ensuring the whole body is working harmoniously together from joints to muscle tissue
- **Physiotherapist**: takes an all-encompassing, science-based approach to physical, psychological and lifestyle aspects of the pain manifestation

Note: if you do decide to try these therapies, it is advisable to check with your rheumatologist prior to treatment. Equally, the treatment is only as effective as the person who is carrying it out, so if a healthcare professional makes you feel uncomfortable or wrongly informs you that they can cure your arthritis – they *may not* be the right person for the job. Check that your practitioner is a registered and qualified professional in their area of expertise.

- **Chiropractic** Spinal manipulation is documented as far back as Hippocrates, but chiropractic was first performed in 1895. It uses manual techniques such as joint adjustment and/or manipulation, with a focus on any dislocation or misalignment of the spine, considered by chiropractors as the root of all ailments. The chiropractic approach regards the body as a whole, whereby a disorder in one part of the neuromusculoskeletal system (meaning the interactions between nerves, muscles and the skeleton) disturbs the rest. Chiropractic treatment has been shown to improve pain, such as joint and back pain, and reduce fatigue.
- **Osteopathy** Regularly confused with chiropractic, osteopathy puts less of an emphasis on the brain and nervous system, with a gentler manipulation and massage of multiple areas. Osteopathy's guiding principle is that the wellbeing of an individual is dependent on the collective interaction between bones, muscles, ligaments, connective tissue and the overall

interrelationship between structure and function. In my experience, an osteopath will adopt a holistic approach, taking the time to understand the wider and patient-specific combination of symptoms, medical history and social factors causing the pain or disturbance in functionality, as opposed to purely concentrating on the site(s) of the problem. The intention is to stimulate the body's own healing properties in a non-invasive way.

As WHO states, osteopathy 'respects the relationship of body, mind and spirit' in health and disease. NICE recommends osteopathy as a possible treatment option for OA, but research thus far is minimal.

- **Physiotherapy** This is a physical therapy that 'helps restore movement and function when someone is affected by injury, illness or disability'. Used with people of all ages with varying health conditions, physiotherapy helps patients through movement and exercise, manual therapy, education and advice on how to improve their condition. While it is a science-based profession, it does navigate pain management with a holistic approach to health and wellbeing, including aspects of a patient's general lifestyle. A physiotherapist may perform exercises *in* the consultation room, but the principal aspect of physiotherapy is patient participation ***outside of it***. You are educated, empowered and supported by a physiotherapist with exercises to use at home, reporting back with progress or limitations.

Physiotherapy is very popular within mainstream medicine and referrals are frequently made by GPs, hospital doctors and surgeons. Successful physiotherapy treatment does rely on the right approach from the therapist, but ultimately it also depends on how much work you put in at home.

- **Occupational therapy** Like physiotherapy, this is a form of rehabilitative care, improving or preventing the worsening of a condition, enabling people to live better alongside their condition, more independently and productively. The therapy has a focus on self-management, aiding patients to develop the skills needed to complete general everyday activities and/or find alternative ways to achieve them with greater independence, whether at home, in social settings or in the workplace. A personalised plan with pain-management and relaxation techniques may be devised, and psycho-social support may also be provided with education or advice around fertility, pregnancy, childcare, work, sex and driving. Being newly diagnosed with arthritis can bring its challenges, and occupational therapy may offer ways to support you or your family, with managing your pain and condition from day to day.
- **Podiatry** A podiatrist is a doctor who specialises in feet and may also be called a doctor of podiatric medicine or DPM. Generally speaking, they are experts in all kinds of pain or injuries in any (and all) parts of the foot, identifying, diagnosing and treating disorders, diseases and deformities of the feet and legs to implement the right care. Podiatrists may assess blood flow, the way you walk and your shoes, providing advice, special footwear or inserts or appropriate exercises.

Tips From Steve

- Sleep, diet, stress, traumatic life events all affect the pain experience, so anything you can do to de-stress, such as sleeping and eating well, movement and exercise, being around people and family you trust and eating as healthily as you can are paramount.
- Feeling helpless and alone is common when living with chronic pain, as it often strips us of our identity. Sharing and finding a community can be the first step to coming out of the isolation of living with chronic pain.
- Finding ways of doing things, however 'small', will be big victories in being able to feel like you have a hold over your pain. There is always something you can do. Anything that promotes a sense of safety and agency inside of you has the potential to reduce your pain manifestation – even something as simple as going for a short walk or making a cup of tea.
- Be mindful and pay attention to the experience in your body.

*

It has taken time to get here, but my hills are a little smaller now. I stand on top of them for a whole while longer and I have a reasonable measure of time before I'm on to another. Something I have learned is that my pain is never separate from me or restricted to the physical area on my body where I am feeling it. It is intrinsically linked to everything else that is happening physically, psychologically and emotionally in my mind and body on that day, or even that week.

As we've explored, the 'pain experience' is more than the physical feeling and sensation of pain. Hopefully, this chapter has provided you with a combination of pain relievers that work for you. After all, your unique pain deserves a unique pain-relief package.

7

Make A Move

'When it comes to health and wellbeing, regular exercise is about as close to a magic potion as you can get.'
Thích Nhất Hạnh, spiritual leader, poet

If someone had told me ten or 15 years ago that at some point in the future I'd be writing a book with a chapter dedicated to exercise, I probably would have chortled uncomfortably and been a little flummoxed. Me? Writing about exercise? You have *got* to be kidding. The last to be selected for a team in PE lessons by my classmates (and even then only because they had no other option), I can grudgingly remember being the person people always avoided passing the ball to, and the one who had zero knowledge about sport. Zilch. Nada.

Exercise back then (and still today) was an activity I enjoyed in solitude. As a young adult, I would grab my iPod Nano and *ir*regularly go on 5k runs around our village, or I would go swimming. Our dad instilled in both my sister and me from a pre-school age that swimming was an essential life skill, and he lovingly dedicated every Saturday morning to taking us to lessons. At university, the theme continued: long jogs around the beautiful 560-acre campus parkland, and swimming in the campus leisure-centre pool. Gyms, to me, were for fitness fanatics or professional weightlifters, and I had no interest in setting foot in one. In fact, I didn't do so until my early 20s; YouTube videos or fitness DVDs were my classes of choice.

Why am I telling you all of this? *Well*, because this chapter is not to tell you to go to the gym, join a netball club or run 5k every day – unless you want to and feel you can. Exercise is personal – always. So, while this chapter is intended to help you on your way to exercising and feeling better in your bones, do it in your own style and at your own pace. And this style and pace could change from day to day, or from year to year. I may not jog as much now, but I do walk. My at-home fitness films are gathering dust, but my yoga mat is out more than it is folded up. And I swim when I have the time.

There is a saying, that you may have heard: 'If you freeze, you seize'. And there may be some truth in this. So, it doesn't matter how, where or when you exercise, just so long as you do some form of it daily. Eighty-one per cent of the Arthritis Foodie community who answered an Instagram poll in August 2020 said that they felt better after exercising, and 82 per cent exercise once a week or more. I appreciate that – generally speaking – because of symptoms such as pain, impaired mobility and fatigue, most people living with chronic conditions tend to exercise less; but it can actually make symptoms worse. Our bodies need movement, and the lack of it results in muscle wasting, poor joint health, reduced fitness and exercise tolerance, a decrease in range of movement and flexibility, as well as a higher risk of other injuries due to poor joint stability.

The positive benefits of movement outweigh not moving. A tsunami of research papers demonstrate that humans function better with movement. Long-term data consistently shows that exercise is much better than brain training or food, and as good as social interaction – it is predictive of living a healthier, happier and longer life. And, as well as the wealth of positive effects on mental health and wellbeing, exercise may also have a positive impact on our gut bugs and microbiome. More human trials are required in this area, but exercise may, in the future, provide a beneficial treatment for several chronic and immune-based diseases.

Exercise and Inflammation

The word 'arthritis', whether you are living with the condition or not, conjures up images of brittle bones, swollen joints, 'bones rubbing on bones', walking sticks and wheelchairs. Whether your arthritis is currently manageable or severe, these thoughts can be difficult to overcome. Exercising might be painful when you live with arthritis, and there may be a niggling fear that you are going to 'make things worse'. But the pain you feel during or after exercise is a small, temporary penance for a better state of long-term physical and mental wellbeing.

As we have learned, inflammation is probably one of the bigger consistent contributors to pain and it's a leading character in the story of chronic inflammatory diseases like arthritis. While overtraining or overexercising can be pro-inflammatory, I have a sense that most of us living with chronic conditions may not be at risk of overexerting ourselves in the way that a professional athlete might.

What we may be at risk of, however, is not moving at all, which can be just as inflammatory as overdoing it. Avoiding the extremes – there is a sweet spot in the middle – has beneficial anti-inflammatory effects. And the dose of movement that people need is surprisingly small.

- Do you need to run a marathon? No.
- Do you have to pay a £40-a-month gym membership? No.
- Do you have to go to a costly workout class three times a week? No.

A recent study has found that just one 20-minute session of moderate exercise can act as an anti-inflammatory, and it costs nothing but your time. So much so that physical activity is now advocated as an anti-inflammatory therapy for patients with rheumatic diseases.

Sedentary behaviour (simply defined as too much sitting) and obesity are associated with a pro-inflammatory status and low-grade inflammation. It has been demonstrated specifically in RA that obesity is associated with higher markers of inflammation. Equally, replacing a sedentary behaviour pattern with increased levels of light, moderate and vigorous activity is accompanied by low inflammatory markers.

Getting Physical with Arthritis

Exercise can bring discomfort, and most people know that if it is not hurting, even a bit (with or without arthritis), their muscles probably are not working hard enough. Your muscles should feel like they have worked and have stretched, but you should not be overly exhausted or in agony. So, some pain is good, but it is essential that you listen to your body.

On the days when you find your body in a flare, with swollen joints, pain, exhaustion and low energy – when it feels like it would be too much – then it *might just be too much*. In this instance, it is best to completely rest and recuperate, exercising when the pain has eased off or choosing a gentle way of exercising if you can manage it. You have to simply do what you can, when you can, and go at your own pace. And remember: comparison is the thief of joy.. So, stop comparing yourself to pro-fitness models on social media (unfollowing them will help) and find joy in your own movement, feeling good in *your* body (you only have one).

Those living with RA who are physically active have been shown to have a milder disease progression and it has been established consistently that exercise has numerous health benefits for RA patients, improving joint health, physical function, mobility and psychological wellbeing, as well as reducing fatigue without aggravating symptoms or inducing further joint damage.

Data indicates that range-of-motion, strengthening and aerobic exercises are all safe and should be included in the overall treatment of those living with conditions such as OA, RA, AS or other diseases involving chronic inflammation. Both aerobic and resistance training can improve physical capacity, muscle function and several clinical symptoms in patients with autoimmune rheumatic diseases, counteracting and reducing inflammation.

MYTH-BUSTER: WHY RUNNING IS NOT BAD FOR YOUR KNEES

People often say that 'running is bad for your knees' or that it can cause knee OA. However, doctors now realise that this is not true and, *when done carefully*, running can actually reduce the pain associated with arthritis. Chiropractor Steve Haines notes consistent data revealing that runners have healthier backs and knees than non-runners. And the benefits of running, even in those with pre-existing conditions such as arthritis, will help people to cope with them. Data show that when you move more and regularly, alongside a reduction in pain and stiffness, your joint cartilage is healthier in the long term, and regular running may, in fact, have a protective effect against the development of OA.

Exercise and You

What, how, where, when . . . we all have to start somewhere with exercise.

As prescribed by many healthcare professionals, we should all aim to be active every day. But exercise does not necessarily mean deadlifting at the gym or doing a hundred press-ups – you have to modify it based on your body, abilities, goals and time. Knowing these is essential because they are different for everyone. While some of us living with arthritis may be able to run a marathon or walk 10,000 steps daily, others may find that a slow mooch outside and back again for ten minutes is challenge enough to begin with. If you are unsure, talk to your rheumatologist or a physiotherapist for advice on exercising safely, but I hope that the following tips will be useful.

The 2018 European League Against Rheumatism's (EULAR) 'Recommendations for Physical Activity in People with Inflammatory Arthritis and Osteoarthritis' has provided us with the first evidence-based guidelines about the quality and quantity of exercise that are beneficial specifically for people living with arthritis. The EULAR recommends regular participation in the following:

- ✓ **Cardiorespiratory (aerobic):** 30–60 minutes per day (a minimum of 150 minutes per week) of purposeful moderate or 20–60 minutes per day (a minimum of 75 minutes per week) of vigorous exercise, or some combination of these
- ✓ **Resistance (strength):** 2–3 days per week training each major muscle group on strengthening activities (legs, hips, back, abdomen, chest, shoulders and arms)

✓ **Range-of-motion (flexibility):** 2–3 days per week stretching major muscle groups
✓ **Neuromotor (balance):** 20–30 minutes on ≥2–3 days/week practising balance
✓ **Reducing any time spent sitting or lying down:** as much as you can, break up long periods of not moving with activity – even if it's small

For reference, 'moderate' activity will raise your heart rate, make you breathe faster and feel warmer – a test is to see if you can still talk, but not sing during the activity. During light activities and strengthening exercises you may be able to still hold a conversation, but during 'vigorous' activity, you will probably not be able to say more than a few words without pausing for breath.

RA may accelerate the loss of muscle mass that typically occurs as people get older, which is why it is important to do exercises that will build muscle, in addition to aerobic exercises that improve the fitness of your heart and lungs. As well as the benefits already discussed, the anti-inflammatory effects of exercise can also reduce stress, fatigue and symptoms of depression, along with plenty of other conditions associated with inflammation. And for everyone, exercise also improves sleep, energy levels, self-esteem, mood and general mental wellbeing. Remember, 20 minutes of moderate activity is the aim to get the anti-inflammatory response.

Light physical activity
• A gentle walk
• Day-to-day housework
• Cooking

Moderate physical activity
• Brisk walking
• Dancing
• Cycling gently, static or on level ground
• Gentle, moderate swimming
• Water aerobics
• Badminton
• Walking or jogging on a treadmill
• Pushing a lawnmower
• Painting and decorating
• Heavy gardening or housework
• Handwashing a car
If you are unable to use your legs and rely on aids, you can achieve moderately intense exercise by using a manual wheelchair or a handcycle (ergometer). Swimming or water aerobics might be helpful too, as well as range-of-motion exercises and chair-based yoga.
Vigorous physical activity
• Jogging or running
• Swimming fast
• Cycling fast or on hills
• Sports such as football, rugby, netball and hockey
• Singles' tennis
Very vigorous activities might be lifting heavy weights, circuit training, sprinting up hills, interval running and spinning classes.

Recommendations Before Starting

Gyms with intimidating equipment, exercise classes full of people with perfect physiques, YouTube videos with exercise enthusiasts talking without any trouble on their 5,000th burpee, yogis doing effortless handstands and bending like elastic . . . It can feel tiring just watching exercise, let alone going and doing it for yourself. So, where do you start?

Well, firstly, I do not know you as well as *you* know you. Neither do the exercise experts on- or offline. Only you know how your body is feeling, the kind of day or week you have had, your pain levels and fitness abilities. You are not going to miraculously morph into Joe Wicks the moment you begin to exercise. And hey, *that's okay*. Exercise does not have to be picture-perfect; you do not need to fixate on duplicating the immaculate moves of fitness professionals. My downward-facing dog was more like a sideward-grappling goat at first – far from steady, with limbs all over the place. But we all have to start somewhere, and not being 'perfect' (whatever 'perfect' is) should not deter you from trying and trying again. Doing something imperfectly (*but not unsafely*) is better than doing nothing at all.

Be cautious

To reiterate: perfection is not the aim. But it is still important to be comfortable and safe when exercising. Exercise in a way that is right for you. If you are a little uncertain about a particular type of exercise and cannot get what you need from a YouTube video, then it might be an idea to take a class or two to learn the moves safely, before doing it at home or by yourself. Perhaps arrive a little earlier to have a conversation with the class instructor, and:

- let them know about your condition
- explain that you may need to go at your own pace and/or
- modify the moves if/when you need to.

Most instructors will thank you for letting them know and come over to support you during the class if needed. I have often raised my hand in a yoga class, and the teacher has kindly helped me to alter the pose until I feel more comfortable.

Alternatively, if you have the financial capacity, consult a professional such as a physiotherapist or a personal trainer who can advise on the best way to exercise for *your* body. They may suggest specific exercises for target areas where you require better range of movement in your joints, or more muscular strength to support them.

Know your pain

As much as exercise is supposed to be slightly painful, it is not meant to make you feel like you have been in a tumble dryer, hit by a bus or set on fire internally. Ensure that you stay aware of how you are feeling before, during and after exercise. Monitor your progress and which forms of exercise you enjoy or, conversely, would rather not do again. Armed with this information, you can adjust when, where and how you exercise next time, and customise it to your ability and pain levels. On the following page (p. 201) you'll find a template exercise tracker to use at home.

Exercise Tracker

1 = low or no pain at all
5 = bearable pain
10 = high pain levels

Date	Description of Exercise	Type of Exercise: Moderate (M) Vigorous (V) Strengthening (S)	Duration of Exercise	How did the exercise make you feel?	Pain Levels (1 to 10)			
					Before	During	Straight After	Day After
23.08. 2020	Fast paced and brisk walk in the park	M	30 minutes	Good	5	4	5	6

A printable version of this and the Trigger Tracker from Chapter 4 are available on my website for you to download.

Be kind to yourself

We all could do with more of this. Setting your goals really high for exercise and not achieving them can feel disheartening. But the very fact that you are making the effort to exercise, and you *are* exercising, demonstrates that you have not failed at all. You are there. You are trying. You are making the time to better your body and your mind. So, try not to be hard on yourself.

The more you exercise, the better you will understand your own body's capabilities and you will know your body enough to set more achievable, reasonable and kinder goals. Using the tracker above, you can really check in with yourself as to what exercise is working for you and what isn't. And over time, this may change too:

- *Feeling bored of the same walk around the block?* Catch a bus and try a different park.
- *Never tried Pilates before? Or yoga?* Book a class and give it a go.
- *Struggling to find the motivation to exercise in or out of home?* Ask someone to join you.

By trying new activities and ways of exercising, you will find something you really enjoy and will be more likely to stick at it, improve your skills and feel good.

EXERCISE TIMELINE

- Ensure you warm up, gently stretch and loosen your body before getting into the exercise. If you have eaten a main meal, make sure to exercise three hours afterwards. If you have not eaten, have a light snack an hour before, ideally one that contains some protein, and is higher in carbohydrate and lower in fat. Hydrate too with plenty of water, and try to avoid anything that dehydrates, such as caffeine or alcohol.
- During stay hydrated, be present in the moment and aware of your whole body. Frequently check in with yourself and how you are feeling. Do not push yourself if you cannot manage it, and do not attempt to force your body into a pose or an exercise that you are unsure of or that brings you severe discomfort.
- Make sure to stretch straight afterwards when cooling down. Another recommendation would be to use a foam roller (a lightweight cylindrical tube coated with ridged foam). This can help to relieve muscle tightness, soreness and inflammation, and increase your joints' range of motion. You could even use a foam roller before exercising, in preparation. Keep hydrated, and if you have not eaten, eat a wholesome meal – but of course, not too close to your bedtime if you've exercised in the evening.

Get Your Body Moving – Any Way You Can

The key exercises to be aware of are range-of-motion, strengthening and aerobic, from light to moderate or vigorous in intensity.

- **Strengthening activities** are focused on the muscles, and are a necessary component to building and maintaining strong bones.
- **Range-of-motion exercises** improve joint function by assisting you in moving each joint through its full range of motion, keeping joints flexible, reducing pain and improving balance and strength.
- **Aerobic physical activity** helps to protect and uphold heart, lung and circulatory health, alongside enhancing mental wellbeing and helping you to maintain a healthy body weight.

Exercise intensity is subjective – what is moderate to one person might be vigorous to someone else. It all depends on how physically fit you are, your abilities and overall health. As mentioned, you know yourself better than anyone else. Depending on your ability, overall health and condition, some of the activities below may be doable and others may not. Pick out the ones that you feel most comfortable trying initially.

Note: it may be advisable to talk to your doctor, physiotherapist or rheumatologist before beginning a new activity that you have not tried before.

Strength, flexibility and balance

- Yoga, tai chi or Pilates
- Lifting weights

- Working with resistance bands
- Doing exercises that use your own body weight, such as push-ups, sit-ups, lunges or squats
- Heavier gardening, such as digging, lifting and shovelling
- Picking up and carrying heavy loads (this may include children)

Range-of-motion and stretching

These exercises include gentle stretching and movements that take joints through their full range of movement. Stretching before and after exercise is a really important part of taking care of your muscular and joint health, reducing any injuries. It is worth being aware of stretching safely and comfortably, rather than overstretching.

Below are some activities that I have learned and use myself, and you may find them relevant to your condition. I have explained one round of movement per exercise, but you can repeat each of them 10 or more times, or for as many minutes as you have time for.

Note: if you have any concerns (such as if you have had surgery or have suffered an injury), please consult your doctor first.

Hands, fingers and thumbs

Place your hands in front of you, either sitting on a chair at a table, on the floor, on an exercise mat or standing at a counter. You can exercise both hands at the same time, or one at a time.

- **Reaching hands** Gently stretch out your whole hand as wide as you are able to, then relax it. Make a tight fist with your thumb on top of your fingers, open and loosen it. Repeat, and repeat on the other side.

- **Travelling fingers** Open your hand out in front of you (palms down on a table might help for stability) and stretch your fingers out away from one another, as far as they can go, like they have had a bad argument; then bring them back together, like they've resolved their quarrel!
- **Thumb rests** Open your hand palm-up and rest your thumb across the palm, then move it out to the side and repeat. Roll and rotate too, if it feels good to do so.
- **Finger pads** Palms up, move your fingertips towards the inner pad of your thumb, touching the area, one fingertip at a time. If this is too difficult, stretch your fingertips to the centre of the palm of your hand instead.

Knees and hips

Start these exercises lying face-up on your back, on an exercise or yoga mat or, alternatively, on your bed. Props can be used to support your knees or lower back (such as cushions, pillows or bolsters). Remember to return to a still position (savasana) between exercises.

- **Hug hold** Stretch your body out and then relax. Bending and bringing your knees towards you and as close to your chest as you can, hug them to you, then let them return back against the floor. You can also do this one leg at a time.
- **Side to side** Move one leg out to the side flat against the floor, as far as it will go, and then return it to its starting position next to the leg that has remained stationary. Swap sides and repeat.

- **In, out, shake it all about:**
  - o **Hips** Sit upright and bring the soles of your feet together as far as you can, making a diamond shape (support your knees with props or cushions if you need to). Move to lie backwards (place a long pillow at the base of your lower back to lie back on if you need to). Place your arms by your sides. This is a 'Reclined Butterfly Pose' in yoga.
  - o **Knees** Lying on your back, bend one knee and keep your foot flat against the floor, sliding it as close as you can to your lower body (or bottom). Then slide your foot back to where it came from and repeat on the other side.
  - o **Legs** Lie with your legs flat against the floor and rotate them in opposite directions outwards, so that your toes are drawn away from one another. Gently shake or wiggle, then rotate your legs in the other direction, both turning in, so that your toes are drawn towards each other like magnets.

Ankles and feet

Sit on the edge of your bed or in a chair, wherever you feel most comfortable, and relax your whole body before starting. What is your face doing? Don't look so anxious! Smile – this is your gift to you today. Isn't it lovely?

- **Rolling and rotating:**
  - o Slightly raise your foot, roll your ankle clockwise in a circle, then anti-clockwise. Swap sides and repeat.
- **Angular stretching:**
  - o **Up/down:** slightly raise your foot and then tilt it (and your toes) towards you, then away from you, as far as it can go each way. Swap sides and repeat.

  - o **Left/right:** with your foot raised, tilt the angle of your foot from left to right, as far as it will go (this one may feel uncomfortable at first). Swap sides and repeat.

These two stretches can be done effectively with your wrists too.

- **Toe-curling stretches:** curl your toes downwards, straighten, then lift. Swap sides. Spread your toes apart and then back together again. Swap sides.

Ask the Expert

For the next part of this chapter I have teamed up with Zoe McKenzie, qualified physiotherapist, personal trainer, Pilates instructor and founder of the blog Actively Autoimmune. Zoe has six years' clinical experience in geriatrics, musculoskeletal conditions, orthopaedics, women's health and working with people who are living with chronic illnesses and health conditions.

Best exercises for core stability and strength at home

The following activities engage your core abdominal muscles, which are really important in stabilising your pelvis and spine. These 'core' muscles work to provide support for every movement, but if any of them is weakened, lengthened, tight or injured, then their *usually* automatic, stabilising action is disrupted. Pain, inflammation and altered movement patterns are all typical in chronic conditions, which will affect how your core works. So, maintaining a strong centre helps to optimise movement throughout your entire body.

Note: use an exercise or yoga mat for the following activities.

Core activation

- You can do this exercise sitting down on a chair, or you can lie on your back on the mat. Place your fingertips on your hip bones. Roll your fingers off the bone and inwards, moving them down slightly into the 'soft' part. Let them sink into the muscle.
- On your next exhale, draw your belly button in towards your spine (you should feel a muscle tightening underneath your fingers).
- Now keep breathing in and out, trying to hold on to this contraction. You should be able to talk and breathe normally while maintaining this. If you can't, you are probably gripping too strongly with your core muscles; the aim is a 4/10 intensity. The rest of your abdominal muscles should be relaxed.

Pelvic tilts

- Ideally, do this exercise sitting down on a chair, or you can lie on your back on the mat. Place your hands on your hips, fingers on hip bones and thumbs on your back.
- Inhale, tilt your pelvis forward, arching your back away.
- Exhale, sitting up straight.
- Then continue. The movement should feel like it is coming from your core rather than tensing your leg muscles.
- Find a balance or middle point between the two, so you find neutral spine (your spine's natural position). Do 5–10 reps.

Knee openings

- Lie on your back, knees bent, neutral spine with core engaged.
- Inhale to prepare.
- Exhale and slowly draw one knee out to the side, keeping the other knee still.
- Inhale. Return the knee back to the centre. Repeat on the other side.

Dead bug

- Lie on your back, knees bent, neutral spine with your core engaged.
- Inhale, float one leg up to 90 degrees at the hip and 90 degrees at the knee, or as far as you can comfortably hold it (but not too high) and leave it there for a moment.
- Exhale to softly lower the leg back down, stretching it out as normal.
- Repeat on the other side.

Bridges

- Lie on your back, knees bent, heels close to your glutes, neutral spine and core engaged.
- Exhale and gently roll the lower back into the mat, then lift your tailbone up towards the ceiling.
- Continue to peel your spine off the mat, bone by bone, until you rest on your shoulder blades. Inhale, and hold.

- Exhale and lower yourself down, drawing your breastbone towards mat and peeling the spine back down, bone by bone, until your tailbone reconnects with the floor and your spine returns to neutral.

*

To finish off, here's a quick Q&A with Zoe:

Q. What if it is too painful?

A. Listen to your body – you know it best. Tune in to how it feels and what it can and cannot tolerate. You may have 'X' condition on paper, but how it presents in you could be completely different to someone else with the same condition. Likewise, how your body responds to exercise will vary based on your exercise tolerance, pain thresholds, how your body manages inflammation and any other conditions you might have. Pain, as discussed in Chapter 6, is an alarm system that can go awry, so your pain may not be indicative of what is actually going on in your body. That being said, it is important to recognise when something may be *too* painful, depending on different scenarios:

- **Acute pain** If it feels sharp or is a new pain in a different area, then stop what you are doing and seek professional advice to find out the cause.
- **Increasing pain in a specific area** This may be the result of not carrying out the prescribed exercises properly, say, by recruiting the wrong muscles that are then being

overloaded, feeding into a pain cycle. Either change exercises, positioning or the intensity of the exercise (resistance, reps, sets) – and if it still it hasn't improved, seek professional advice.

- **Increased pain all over – your usual pain, but worse** It is likely that you have tried to do too much too soon. Rest until your pain levels return to normal, and then try again. But do a lot less – even less than you think you can manage to start with – then check how you feel immediately after, the next day and 2–3 days after as well, to see how your body recovers and tolerates movement. If it all feels okay, then you can gradually increase the time or intensity.

Gym instructors and personal trainers are often not trained to work with people who are living with chronic conditions, so it could be that you have not received the right advice on how to exercise safely with your condition. If you continue to experience difficulties with exercise, speak to your specialist or physiotherapist.

Q. What is the best type/frequency of exercise for chronic conditions?

A. The key to exercising with a chronic illness is finding what suits you, and you have to work with your physiology. Options that work really well with chronic conditions are low-impact resistance strengthening exercises, Pilates, some types of yoga, swimming and static cycling. In general, three to five sessions a week is a good starting point, but this depends on what you are doing and what your exercise tolerance level is. If you are starting exercise again after a long period of being inactive, you want to ease into it slowly, starting with one to three sessions a week to see how your body recovers each time. Little and often might be more suitable. Quality and consistency of movement matter most, rather than quantity. As a guide, for strength training you typically do: 8–12 reps, 1–4 sets, with 2–3-minute rests between sets.

Q. Have people seen a difference in their symptoms after following exercise plans?

A. Common themes in patients with chronic diseases are fatigue, tight muscles, joint pain and stiffness. Exercise plans are personal to them, taking their specific health needs into account. After an assessment, I always start exercises at a low level focusing on the quality of movement, over its quantity or intensity. Reconnecting to our bodies is an important first step for all. It is vital to find a balance and listen to your body, knowing when to rest and when to exercise, working *with* your body rather than against it.

As an example, a client with RA and gastrointestinal issues was unable to exercise and very deconditioned. A simple strengthening exercise programme, in lying or seated positions with short (15–20-minute) but frequent (4–5 times a week) sessions, plus a gentle mobility/stretching programme did not flare their pain, and after their first four weeks they reported feeling stronger and found everyday tasks easier. They also felt a huge sense of accomplishment and more connected to their bodies.

*

Although the thought of – even the word – 'exercise' might seem overwhelming at first, rather than seeing it as a task to be ticked off, an activity you have to do, try to see it as daily movement woven into your schedule – whatever this may look like. And remember, it won't look the same every day, or every week. Some days I can manage a whole hour of yoga, others only ten minutes or none at all. Sometimes I can go for an hour-long walk and other days I can only do 20 minutes around the block. The main thing is to do it.

You will define what exercise is to you, and that definition can change from one day to the next; all that matters is that you feel good doing it. And trust me when I say that you *will* feel happier afterwards (endorphins are released with exercise, so scientifically it really does make you happy) – no matter how big or small the movement, or how long it lasts.

8
Rest and Sleep

'Sleep is that golden chain that ties health and our bodies together.'
Thomas Dekker, Elizabethan dramatist and writer

Are you getting enough sleep? Do you fall asleep at the same time every evening and wake up at roughly the same time every morning? Do you feel rejuvenated when you wake up? Is falling asleep easy for you, or is getting to sleep a conscious nightmare?

Sleep seems to be slipping through our fingers, eluding us more and more, and yet it is as vital to our health as it ever has been. Good, sound sleep is a universal staple to health here on planet earth, and all species need it – or something that appears astonishingly like it – even bees, fish and frogs.

The nature of sleep, from the various stages to its duration, is vastly changeable from species to species. Evolution has equipped dolphins with the capacity to keep one half of their brain wide awake, while the other half slumbers. *Pretty phenomenal.* Sleep is so profoundly essential that we humans spend about a third of our lives doing it – or attempting to, in the case of many of us living with a chronic condition. Sleep is imperative to the health of our brains and bodies, and it even makes our gut bugs happier. Despite its importance, sleep is undervalued throughout much of the Western world, with the WHO describing a 'global epidemic of sleeplessness', noting that roughly two-thirds of adults are sleeping less than the necessary eight hours a night. For some, this is out of choice: they may be glued to a screen streaming a film or responding to emails; for others, it is circumstantial, as children disturb snooze time; and for others still – such as those living with arthritis – chronic pain inhibits their ability to get *to* sleep and/or have a restful slumber.

Catch-22: Painsomnia

Pain induces a lack of sleep and lack of sleep induces pain. Unsurprisingly, sleep disturbances are present in 67–88 per cent of chronic-pain disorders, and according to the Arthritis Foundation, as many as 80 per cent of arthritics have difficulty sleeping. With sore, stiff and swollen joints to contend with, sleep is not as simple as it should be, as we struggle to get comfortable, nod off and stay asleep. We tend to suffer the day after too, unable to function at full capacity because of an overwhelming layer of exhaustion and pain. Everything feels hazy – a sensation that arthritics and other chronic-pain-syndrome sufferers refer to as 'brain fog'. But there may be some science behind this 'brain fog', as memories formed when sleep-deprived are fainter, fading in the hours and days afterwards. British scientist and sleep expert Matthew Walker explored the effect of sleep on the brain's ability to learn new things, discovering that subjects who were sleep-deprived before learning remembered 40 per cent less than those who were not deprived of sleep.

The inability to sleep because of pain has been termed 'painsomnia', and although this is not deemed proper medical terminology, it is a very real phenomenon. Countless times I have been lying in bed feeling exhausted, but frustratingly unable to sleep because of fire-like burning sensations in my ankles or tingling swelling in my fingers. The difficulty of getting to sleep, the fatigue of the disease, layered with one or more poor nights of sleep, results in arthritis seeming (and being) so much worse, creating a vicious cycle that seems impossible to break. And, when you are in this cycle it has a mental hold over you: the more you think about not being able to sleep the more likely you are to, well . . . not sleep!

Pain and sleep are bidirectional, meaning that pain can lead to sleep deprivation and sleep deprivation can lead to pain. In this way, pain can be both a cause and an effect of inadequate sleep. In chronic-pain patients and even in healthy, pain-free individuals, lack of sleep has been shown to contribute to the exacerbation of pain processes. Our understanding of the bidirectional relationship between pain and sleep, although established, is in its infancy and needs to be considered further, not only for the benefit of chronic-pain prevention for people living with conditions such as arthritis, but for the health of the wider public.

Sleep and Immunity

Sleep has numerous benefits for our brains and bodies – so much so that science has yet to find a biological function that does not benefit from a good night's sleep, or suffer without it. Our immunity especially is compromised when we do not clock up our recommended minimum of eight hours a night. Sleep and the immune system are intertwined: sleep fights and protects against all manner of infections when we are well, and the immune system stimulates sleep when we are not. This gives a whole new meaning to the phrase 'sick and tired' – you are tired when you are sick and you are sick when you are tired.

Losing sleep for just one night has a profound and detrimental impact on our immune systems. We all have an army of natural killer cells, powerful participants in the workings of the immune system, and our first-line defence when it comes to identifying and destroying foreign elements, from viruses to cancerous cells. Just one impaired night's sleep reduces this specialised army, and with its battalion depleted, our defences truly are down. Shorter sleep duration has been associated with increased susceptibility to the common cold, resulting in a high infection rate in those who have slept for only five hours or fewer.

If you are living with any chronic autoimmune, inflammatory and pain-inducing condition, it is only to be expected that a whole load more sleep is required (more so than the average person without any such condition), particularly when in the throes of a flare-up that can often feel like you are full of cold. *Ringing true for you*? In my first couple of months living with arthritis I felt staggeringly fatigued. I had to take leave from university for six weeks, during which time I slept for hours in the day and whenever I could at night – sometimes up to 16 hours in all. Every disturbed night's sleep exacerbated (while also being related to) my pain and inflammation, and I desperately required sleep *for* the pain and inflammation too.

Pain, Sleep and Inflammation: They're All Connected

As we discovered in Chapter 6, all pain originates from an inflammatory response. Pain, sleep and inflammation are therefore inextricably linked, and as research in this field develops, it is becoming clearer that the connection between them is multi-directional. Initially, restless nights were deemed an inevitable outcome of living with arthritis, but scientists are confirming that not only does joint pain trigger a loss of sleep, but sleep disturbance worsens joint pain and can even accelerate joint damage.

The circadian rhythm defines the natural, internal biological processes that recur on a daily 24-hour cycle, and inflammation can lead to circadian sleep disorders. Reduced sleep has also been found to substantially increase pro-inflammatory cytokines and inflammation. So it works both ways.

Emerging evidence suggests that when the body is in a fasted state – as it is during sleep – it produces a substance called BHB, which directly interferes with the process of inflammation connected to several disorders, including AIDs and inflammatory conditions. Moreover, sleep is the longest duration that we are able to avoid feeling stressed, and stress too has a profound impact on inflammation, which we will look at in further detail in Chapter 9. So, overall, the sleep–inflammation connection is vital in overcoming a difficult night's sleep and achieving a restful one.

Five Steps to Essential Sleep Hygiene

Now that you are, hopefully, more mindful of the effects that sleep can have on the body when living with arthritis – its connection to immunity, pain and inflammation, and why we require it, but struggle to attain it – how can you improve its duration and quality?

Unfortunately, nobody else can do it for you, but I can provide you with some tools to take away and try, starting with sleep hygiene. No, this does not equate to me telling you to wash your bedding and take a shower – I shall *presume* you already have this covered. Sleep hygiene is, in fact, a variety of recommendations, from day- to night-time habits, devised to promote healthy sleep and full daytime alertness. Originally set out for the treatment of mild to moderate insomnia, the original principles are all here, with a few more thrown in. So, without further ado, I give you your sleep-hygiene tips to integrate into your daily routine.

1. Think of your gut

It is never too long before I bring your awareness back to the gut. The gut never sleeps, but it does benefit from the time when you are asleep or not eating, as we just discovered.

So, how can you give your gut (and therefore your digestion and your sleep) a little help?

- **Leave it alone.** Time without any food interruptions is a start, but if you are munching on a late-evening snack or have consumed a large dinner right before bedtime, that gut of yours won't be getting its required space and respite. Eating at night is typically accompanied by poorer sleep and gastrointestinal reflux, worsening sleep quality and inflammation by inhibiting the anti-inflammatory fasted state. The digestive system needs time to do its job – i.e. to *digest* – so, if you can avoid eating for two to three hours before your regular bedtime, that should aid a better night's sleep. If your gut is peaceful, then hopefully you can be too.
- **Watch the quantity and quality of your food.** How often do you catch yourself grazing throughout the day – whether it is picking away at a box of grapes, making them last a few

hours in the afternoon, or snacking on something sweet to go with a mug of tea? *Don't worry – you are not the only one.* Apparently, we spend up to 16 hours a day frequently and erratically eating, and *I am a self-confessed snackaholic.* Nutritionist Victoria Jain recommends eating quality foods, leaving five hours between each meal and eating within a 10–12-hour window daily – or even less for some people, depending on their nutrition goals – which reduces body weight, increases energy and improves sleep. Giving your digestive system a break with intermittent fasting or fasting regimes also helps to heal the gut and aid cellular regeneration.

- **Step away from the caffeine.** Caffeine is a stimulant, and from an espresso shot to a Yorkshire brew, it is one of sleep's silent nemeses. The sleep-disruptive effects of caffeine have been well researched, and it has even been used in experiments to replicate insomnia. Found naturally in numerous plants and foods, it blocks the sleep-inducing activities in the brain that build up during the day and it increases adrenaline production. When we feel the end of a burst of energy we may assume that the caffeine is out of our systems, and reach for another caffeine 'hit' – *pass me an oak-milk latte.* But despite the effects potentially going unseen, caffeine is still joyriding in the bloodstream and that second dose will be topping it up. The caffeine equivalent to a large shop-bought coffee reduces the duration of sleep significantly, even when taken six hours before bedtime. Refrain from substantial caffeine consumption (around 400mg of caffeine, which is two coffees, depending on their strength) for a minimum of six hours before your head hits the pillow. If you drink a caffeinated coffee at 12pm lunchtime, 12 hours later in bed at midnight, a quarter of the caffeine is still in your brain. So, best advice would be to have only a small amount of caffeine earlier in the day (before 12), in the form of a matcha or a green tea, for instance, and stick to herbal teas thereafter. Sorry, I know this information is the stuff of nightmares!

- **Don't turn to a nightcap for your shut-eye.** 'Just a glass of wine to help me sleep tonight' or 'a little nightcap's' worth of a spirit on ice. The familiar notion that alcohol will send you off into a slumber is a myth. True, it may knock you out if overconsumed, but this is not restorative, regular and essential sleep. Alcohol, unlike caffeine, is a sedative that sedates parts of your brain. But sedation does not equate to the benefits of sleep. The initial sedating effect is short lived, resulting in a fragmented and disturbed sleep in the second part of the night, with the restorative stage of sleep suppressed and an increase in wakefulness. In short, alcohol has a profound impact on sleep, and we have already learned about its other potential effects in Chapter 3.

2. Exercise, but not before bed

Exercise can deepen our sleep, so using the tips from Chapter 7, try to incorporate it into your daily routine. Just 150 minutes of moderate to vigorous activity each week is associated with a 65 per cent improvement in sleep quality – so long as it is not right before bed. Any intense exercise is stimulating for the body and the brain, which can make falling asleep a lot harder. Gentle yoga before sleeping does, however, seem to help me off to a deep slumber: I use 'bedtime' yoga sequences, light candles and massage strained joints with CBD oil to do it.

3. Make the most of the day

Soak up the sunlight. Natural daylight is essential to our body clocks and circadian rhythms. I feel overwhelmingly grateful to have a garden. Bathing in the rays, breathing in the fresh air and basking in nature is an absolute salvation. The more daylight we absorb, the more vitamin D we have to improve our sleep (a number of studies link low levels of vitamin D with sleep disorders, impaired sleep quality and reduced sleep). The majority of us are accustomed to 16 hours of continuous wakefulness and 8 hours of sleep in one 24-hour cycle, but centuries ago, humans made time for a brief nap in the afternoon, and some cultures still make time to do this. So, if you feel yourself falling into a lull in the afternoons, you have your ancestors to blame.

4. Keep to a sleep schedule

Tempting as it may be to nap during the day or bask in a Sunday lie-in, it is still essential to keep to your circadian rhythm, maintaining the same sleep schedules during the weekend as you have implemented in the week. The regularity of going to bed and waking up at the same time each day is a key part of a wholesome good night's rest. Even if you have stayed up later than planned, or if you have had a bad night of sleep, whether it's a weekday or weekend, be sure to wake up at your usual time. You should find that falling asleep and waking up are easier, and that you have an improved circadian rhythm. I know this is easier said than done though, and my mum will be more than happy to remind me of the endless lie-ins I've had over the years. I remember when she used to wake me up at 9am with a mug of tea, which would have been cold by the time I got around to drinking it, at 12 pm. But I do try hard to stick to a routine now, as I know how important it is.

5. Detox on digital devices

Do you scroll through your phone before bed? Watch a film? Catch up on emails on another device? The modern, 24-hour-a-day digital world we find ourselves in – with Smartphones, iPads, Kindles and laptops – leaves many of us anxious to always be 'on'. But isn't it time we switched off sometimes? No, I'm not about to tell you to unplug your WiFi router or swap your smartphone for an analogue dial-up – because technology is a wondrous tool. But that is just it: it is a *tool* that we should be controlling, not the other way round. The hormone melatonin is unable to do its very important daily task of inducing sleep in the presence of too much light, as in the case of our bright-blue-screen electronic devices. Reading an iPad at night suppresses the release of melatonin by more than half, whereas reading a printed book does not suppress it at all.

All-important Sleep Aids

Once you have your sleep hygiene routinely sorted, there are a number of additional ways to change your sleep for the better that are worth trying.

Reduce your stress

As mentioned at the beginning of this chapter, the way that sleep, inflammation and pain are linked is multifaceted. And the way in which we think about both pain and sleep can worsen both, creating a cycle. These negative and stressful thoughts may bombard us during the day and join us in our beds at night. Whether these stressors are triggered within us from our chronic pain, or outside of us, in our lives or work, their impact on our sleep can be detrimental. I find relaxation and methods to reduce pain and quieten the mind really help (see Chapters 6 and 9). Conditions such as back pain, fibromyalgia and arthritis, directly associated with negative thoughts about insomnia and pain, can be effectively managed by cognitive-behavioural therapy (CBT).

Calm cocoon

As well as becoming calm internally, creating calm externally is paramount. Although this might not be doable all the time, the one place that you should try to keep as your sanctuary is your bedroom, reserving it for strictly bedroom activity only. Think about it for a moment: has your once-serene place to rest and recharge turned into a hub of activity, from watching television to working on your laptop? The mental associations we establish with our beds can make it harder to fall asleep, so ensure that these are conducive to a good night's sleep and that the environment around your bed encourages it too. Consider the following:

- **Create comfort.** Invest in a mattress that epitomises comfort. Try to choose one that is supportive, but not too firm. If this is not financially possible for you, then I would recommend a memory-foam topper, which is less expensive than a new mattress and just as good. Of course, this comfort has to extend to other components of your bed too, such as soft bed linen, a suitable pillow, breathable nightwear (or none at all, if you prefer) or even a weighted blanket, as recommended by pharmacist Raj Vara. Also known as a therapeutic/pressure/gravity blanket, this creates a sense of being swaddled, providing warmth and security, inducing the body to relax. When using a weighted blanket, people with insomnia appear to have a calmer night's sleep. Another practical idea is to use multiple pillows strategically to support problem joints, either as extra padding or to raise them higher. Getting cosy under the sheets, but keeping the room temperature cool is also helpful for getting those 40 winks.

- **Find comfort in the darkness.** It probably goes without saying, but I will say it anyway: you need to eliminate all noise and light to aid the release of melatonin and have a restful sleep. Sleep was a huge struggle for me at university, as I lived in a flat on campus with 12 other people . . . yes, 12! And when I fell poorly (and before my mum took me home), I did have to try and manage some form of sleep, during the day and night, as I was so fatigued. My two saviours were my eye mask and my foam earplugs. So, if you are finding it hard to fall asleep – and stay asleep – these are things that you could try. Fortunately, my student room had blackout blinds, which helped tremendously, and if you can afford to fit these in your bedroom, I would recommend doing so.
- **Test your inner alarm clock.** Something else noise-related is the dreaded alarm clock. But the more aligned you become with your circadian rhythm, waking up and falling asleep at

> the same time each day, the less likely you may be to need one. When I am accustomed to, and sticking to, my wake/sleep schedule, I find myself waking up five minutes before my alarm clock to turn it off. Waking up naturally is far gentler on the body, and by maintaining a routine you may be able to prime your internal clock, subliminally telling yourself to wake at a certain time.

With modern-day hoops to jump through, shift work or other reasons to wake up at specific times, such as a train to catch or a meeting to get to, it is not always possible to avoid the use of an alarm clock. But its sudden shriek might be damaging to our health and our already stressed and inflamed bodies. A light-based alarm clock is a more natural alternative to a sound-based one, as the human body is sensitive to light and dark when it comes to sleep, but you may have to ditch the eye mask to get the full benefit.

Setting yourself up for sleep

If you are to avoid caffeine, the traditional 'nightcap' and any midnight snacks, what are the alternatives to send you to the land of Nod? Here is what I do – or try to do – to cultivate the best kind of sleep:

Every night:

- No drinking liquids (if I can help it) at least two hours before I go to sleep – so if I have a calming tea or hot cacao, it never comes with me to bed.

- I aim for the temperature to be comfortably cool. I usually sleep with the window slightly ajar to let the air flow too (more so in the summer).
- My phone is set to 'night mode', which routinely silences all notifications from 9pm until 8am the next day. I have placed selected contacts on the 'emergency' list, however; so, if my mum calls, for example, she would be able to get through.
- From 7pm to 9am my phone/laptop/iPad are on 'night light' automatically, changing the light from blue to orange, so they no longer emit blue (melatonin-reducing) light. I also reduce the brightness of my devices an hour or so before bed and try to refrain from using them.
- I read a chapter of a book, always in paperback and not via my phone or iPad, ensuring my body is not prevented from producing exactly what it needs for a quality night of rest.
- The light is dimmed in my bedroom and in the rest of the house, wherever possible, before I go to bed.
- I keep a notebook or pad and pen next to my bed, so that if I am struggling to sleep because I am thinking about what I need to do tomorrow (or have not done that day), I simply write it down.
- I try mindfulness methods and list happy moments – whether mentally or in writing – to make me feel calm and happy.
- My phone is on charge and far enough away from me that I would have to physically get out of bed to check it. This works – when I am tired and snuggled up, nothing much is moving me.
- If I am failing to sleep, following the box breathing method (see p. 249) is a useful tool to bring awareness and calm back into the body.

Some nights:

- Hot/cold therapy – this can be in the form of heat wraps (heated in the microwave) or ice packs. Use these for as long as you need. I heat my wraps, then put socks on and lay them over my socks on my ankles. This is important, as I got rashes after going to sleep with these on without socks!
- A hot bath – as soon as you step out of it, there is likely to be a dip in your body temperature to match the temperature of the room, aiding a restful sleep.
- Bedtime yoga – there are some wonderful sequences on YouTube that do seem to send me off to sleep nicely. I do these before reading for a while in bed though, giving me enough time away from the screen before my head hits the pillow.
- Meditation and mindfulness – some tips on the benefits of doing this and how to do it are in the next chapter (see pp. 240–2).

During the day:

- Blue-light-blocking glasses really help me and have reduced the frequency and intensity of my screen-induced headaches.

Helpful Herbs and Edibles for Exhaustion

Equipped with the pain remedies in Chapter 6, gentle exercise in Chapter 7 and mindfulness in Chapter 9, you should be well set up for getting your sleep into a better place. But as we all know, arthritis doesn't make sleep too easy, so I have included some additional remedies here for a good night's sleep, including melatonin-inducing foods and herbal teas.

Foods for sleeping soundly

- **Melatonin** is produced by our bodies to regulate our sleep–wake cycles, signaling to our brains that it is time to sleep. But it can also be found naturally in certain plant-based foods such as pistachios, almonds, black pepper, wholegrains such as oats or brown and black rice, kidney beans, lentils and mushrooms.
- **Tryptophan** cannot be made by the body, so we have to consume foods that contain it, so our bodies can turn it into a B vitamin called niacin. (Niacin plays a key role in creating serotonin, associated with sleep and melatonin levels, to aid in inducing sleep.) Found in a wide variety of protein-containing foods such as eggs, cheese, meat and poultry, fish, rice, and bananas.

Try a tea – the herbal kind

Just as a hot bath can cool you down for sleep, a hot herbal tea can do the same. It seems counterintuitive, but science informs us that this is, in fact, the best way to cool down, and as previously mentioned, the cooler we are, the more likely we are to fall asleep. But remember, no drinking within two hours of bedtime, if you can help it.

- **Chamomile** Derived from dried daisy-like flowers, chamomile has an earthy, yet sweet taste, and it pairs well (or is often found with) honey. It is an ancient medicinal herb, containing a wealth of phytonutrients in the form of flavonoids, and it may be anti-inflammatory and promote sleepiness. It is widely regarded as a 'mild tranquilliser' and 'sleep-inducer', shown to enhance the quality of sleep, alleviate depression and even cause people to fall asleep 15 minutes faster.

- **Valerian root** An extract of the root of valerian, a plant with small, clustering white flowers, this has been extensively used to treat sleeping disorders in Europe for decades. Valerian before bedtime may improve sleep quality, but more studies are needed. It can be taken as a tea, or as a supplement (between 300 and 400mg, 30–60 minutes before bedtime).
- **Passion flower (or *Passiflora incarnata*)** There are about 500 known species of passion flower, and it has been linked traditionally to treating anxiety and sleep disturbance. In one trial, participants consumed a daily dose of passion-flower or a placebo tea. After seven days, those who had drunk the passion-flower tea described improvements in sleep quality. According to some studies, it functions by increasing the naturally occurring amino acid gamma-aminobutyric acid (GABA) in the brain, producing a calming sedative effect, relieving anxiety, enhancing mood and promoting sleep. If you want to get a calming GABA effect into your day (lunchtime) it can be found naturally in varieties of green, black and oolong tea, as well as in fermented foods including kefir, yoghurt and tempeh.
- **Lemon balm** A lemon-scented herb belonging to the same family as mint, lemon balm has been used since as long ago as the Middle Ages to reduce stress and anxiety, stimulate sleep and ease pain and discomfort from indigestion. While its extract may be used in aromatherapy, its dried leaves can

be used to make tea. One small study showed a significant reduction in symptoms of insomnia, but it was funded by a lemon-balm brand, so further studies are needed. Interestingly though, increases in GABA (see previous entry) with lemon-balm use have been demonstrated.

- **Peppermint** There is not much scientific evidence to suggest that peppermint enhances sleep, but peppermint oil does have the capacity to act as a muscle relaxant, and its therapeutic effects may help you to relax and sleep more peacefully. For more information on peppermint, turn back to p. 176, and also try the recipe for peppermint tea on p. 154.

Some More Slumber Suggestions

Sleeping soundly might seem like something that can only be achieved by the pain-free, stress-free population, but with the tips above and a few more suggestions below, you will be more than equipped to enjoy the fully restorative and restful night's sleep that you deserve – every night.

Lavender

The word may be used to describe both a soft purple colour and the plant with a potent perfume-like aroma, but lavender also has a rich herbal-medicinal history. It can be found in the form of balms, oils, sprays and teas, with many people touting its benefits for sleep and stress. The scent of lavender extract and oil has been shown to stimulate activity in areas of the brain, boosting and improving mood and producing a calming effect in the mind, but it's less clear if lavender tea can offer similar benefits.

My mum uses a lavender spray on her pillow before sleeping (I do too now), and it makes complete sense, as the calming effect of the scent is also thought to promote sleep. As well as pharmacist Raj Vara recommending it to aid sleep, studies have shown significantly better sleep quality after breathing in lavender. Lavender essential oil and tea have also been demonstrated to increase quality of sleep and reduce anxiety levels, fatigue and depression.

Magnesium and essential oils

Two more important additions to your sleep arsenal are magnesium and a range of essential oils. For more detail on these, see the following pages: 39, 40, 174 and 184.

9

Be Kind To Your Mind

> 'The single biggest act of bravery or madness anyone can do is the act of change.'
> *Matt Haig, author*

Mind matters. The mind matters. Evidence has shown its association with the gut, but what about its connection to arthritis and those living with long-term conditions? The burden of pain takes not only a physical toll, but a mental one too. With the chronic nature of our condition, pain leads to social withdrawal and anxiety. Depression is four times more common among people in persistent pain compared to those without pain.

Whether you have had depression or not, the mental struggles of living with a chronic disease are all too common and people with long-term musculoskeletal conditions were shown to be almost twice as likely to report feeling anxious or depressed compared to the rest of the population. I get it. I have been there. And I am still there sometimes. It is not something you should ever have to hide or attempt to 'fix' alone.

Foreseeing a life with arthritis, as well as living with it, can of course be both frustrating and upsetting. But every day that you overcome it, you master a life with it. *And you have to take that wheel* – or the car will drive for you (and probably not very well). It takes time to feel all right about living with arthritis, and it's okay if this doesn't happen right now. But it is exhausting to hide what is happening to you; to pretend everything is 'fine' or 'normal' can feel like a burden, and an added stress that you don't need. If you live with it, you will soon be able to really *live* with it.

Are You Stressed?

Stress is a modern-life human predicament. We all live in our stress more than we care to notice, and it is not only detrimental to our mental health, but also to our overall physical wellbeing. Worrying about getting to an appointment on time, dealing with transport delays or traffic disruption, remembering to pick up your prescription, meeting a deadline at work, finding time to call or visit your grandparents – these are all relatable and real everyday stress inducers (or stressors). Stress can also be the result of bigger traumas – losing someone close to you, your job or home, or waiting for a medical diagnosis. Life comes with its stresses. But stress (like inflammation) is intended to be a temporary state, so when it continues to exist subliminally, it may become detrimental to our health.

But it's not all bad

Not all stress is bad though. You are probably thinking, How can any stress be any good for me? Well, 'good stress' can mean those excited butterflies you feel in your stomach, embarking on a challenge like public speaking or a job interview. It is there for the moment, intended to be short lived, to help us rather than hinder us.

But stress can vary from person to person too. For example, whereas I loved being in school theatre productions my sister was terrified by the mere thought of them. So, one person's 'good stress' can be someone else's 'bad stress'. There is no right or wrong: human stress is varied and personal to the individual.

Over the course of our evolution, humans have used the stress response to manage difficult or potentially dangerous situations, keeping us alert and ready to defend or run, otherwise known as the 'fight-or-flight response'. The stress response is unconsciously triggered by the brain's alarm system and activates the release of the hormones adrenaline and cortisol. Adrenaline raises the rate of our heart and breathing, preparing our muscles for action, giving us that 'rush' feeling. Cortisol is the main stress hormone that dampens down our immune system and restrains any bodily functions that are deemed non-essential in a high-stress situation.

Substantial evidence indicates that stress activates the inflammatory response in, and outside of, the brain. Acute experiences of stress appear to enhance immune function, whereas chronic stressors are suppressive. Accumulating research indicates that excessive inflammation plays a critical role in the relationship between stress and stress-related diseases.

Chronic Stress: Chronic Inflammation

As we know, the inflammatory response is intended to be short-lived and temporary, and so is stress: once the 'threat' has passed, your body is supposed to return to normal following the acute stress response. But severe, acute stress, such as near-death experiences or assaults, can lead to mental-health issues and may also worsen into a chronic state of stress. Developing research indicates how elevated levels of social stress can increase bodily inflammation, with new evidence showing that people who have had traumatic experiences in childhood are more likely to be inflamed as children and adults. Chronic psychological stress is connected with the body losing its ability to regulate the inflammatory response, which can then promote the development and progression of certain diseases. Again, this makes me wonder if the loss of my father in childhood impacted the onset of my arthritis.

So, if your body is living with a chronic inflammatory condition, any stress may intensify this inflammation. As mentioned, I find that my joints swell and my pain levels skyrocket when I'm stressed. It is no coincidence that your symptoms are – and feel – worse when you are stressed. And an inflamed body is an inflamed mind. Despite current mainstream medicine largely still treating the body and mind as separate entities, they are undeniably intertwined, and breakthrough new science from pioneering neurologists is overturning the previous way of thinking. Your body may be what you see in the mirror, but a whole world lies within.

Over the last ten years, it has become clear that inflammatory cytokines in the blood can send signals across the blood–brain barrier (BBB), from the body to the brain, causing the mind to become inflamed. When healthy individuals were given a vaccine that spiked inflammation and cytokine levels, there was a sickness-associated mood change and depression. Similarly, those living with chronic inflammatory diseases are often accompanied by depressive symptoms, which, once thought of as an emotional affliction of their condition, is seemingly more likely to be a physiological symptom of it. A radically better way of treatment would be to deal with mental and physical disorders together, rather than separately (as we currently do). In fact, there is some innovative new research that is considering anti-inflammatory agents to treat depression.

The Gut: Food and Mood

Groundbreaking investigations following the effects of inflammation on the brain is being accompanied by progressive research in the sphere of the gut–brain connection and the role of psychobiotics.

'Psychobiotics' is a term coined by neuropharmacologist John Cryan and psychiatrist Ted Dinan to describe live organisms that, when ingested in adequate amounts, work on the gut–brain connection to alleviate symptoms for sufferers of conditions including depression, IBS and chronic fatigue.

Research indicates that the gut influences our feelings and communicates with the brain. Antioxidant-rich foods (as described in Chapter 2) have been shown to lower the risks of depression and cognitive decline, while people who consume an inflammatory diet have a 40 per cent greater risk of depression. There is a proven direct connection between a poor diet and depression and anxiety. An inadequate mix of microbes in the gut microbiome can disrupt the immune system and raise inflammation, which means that there is the potential for psychobiotics to be used as stress management. We are only just beginning to fully realise the importance of gut function and the food we eat to our mental wellbeing.

Communication is Key

Saying yes when you should be saying no? Or, saying no when you should be saying yes? Almost half of people living with arthritis avoid making plans. Setting boundaries, saying no when you need to and taking time to recuperate and rest are vital. Never feel guilty for putting your needs first and taking care of you. But note also that consistently saying no could leave you feeling more isolated. Lack of social contact has profound effects on our minds, bodies and immunity, because we are naturally social creatures. Dr Micah and chiropractor Steve Haines previously mentioned the importance of emotional wellbeing and healthy relationships (see p. viii and p. 189). But if your condition means that you really cannot leave the house at this moment in time, then I also have some suggestions that may help you to feel less alone and isolated (see 'Safe Spaces', pp. 251–2).

Mind–body Therapies

Therapies for listening to (and becoming attuned to) your mind and body . . . I sense an eye-roll here. But this is not a yoga-is-going-to-cure-you moment, and I am not about to tell you to meditate away your arthritis. For the longest time though, I did not listen to my mind or my body nearly half as much as I do now. I thought that taking the time to be mindful would be using up time allocated to something 'more important', and that it would be *a waste* of time.

But mind–body therapies are not a load of nonsense; rather, they are go-to solutions *because they actually work*. Chi, qigong, yoga and meditation actually provide consistent reductions in certain markers of inflammation and can improve symptoms of depression and anxiety. Rheumatologist Lauren Freid says that one of the top things she recommends to her patients is starting and developing a regular yoga or mind–body movement practice. The mind–body connection can help to shift focus and reduce the experience and perception of physical pain.

Buddhist tradition holds that when one person is touched with the feeling of pain they may feel two pains: physical and mental; yet when another is touched by the same pain, they may feel only the physical sensation, and not be affected by it mentally – so they feel only one pain. You are allowed to be upset, disappointed and sad; suppressing these feelings will not help, but being mindful of them will. Unpicking the grief that you may feel at your diagnosis, accepting it and moving forward (not moving on) with it will feel much lighter.

Was I heartbroken at the passing of my wonderful dad? Yes. Was I a crying, snotty mess at finding out I had arthritis and would have to be on a chemotherapy-based drug? Yes. I felt all of it. Do I choose to sit and wallow in the sadness of these feelings every minute of every day? No. Pain from our arthritis is an experience, and suffering is the reaction to this experience – an emotional reaction that we may be able to (sometimes) control, versus the physical reality of the pain we may not always have reign over. Recognising your pain, understanding it, acknowledging it, but not becoming it, underpins the following methods.

Staying in the moment with mindfulness

How many times have you arrived somewhere, but cannot remember how you got there? Have you ever eaten your dinner, then looked down to discover that your plate is empty? Either distracted (by your phone, the TV or someone talking to you), daydreaming or entering into an unconscious 'autopilot' mode – we all do it. Well, mindfulness is the opposite of this.

Defined as 'the practice of being aware of your body, mind and feelings in the present moment' to 'create a feeling of calm', mindfulness is not a new concept. A feature of the 2,500-year-old tradition of Buddhist psychology and thought, it has been modified for use in mental-health psychotherapies with profound effects on overall wellbeing, chronic pain, anxiety and depression. Mindfulness is simple enough to be practised every day and is a form of meditation.

With committed practice to becoming more aware, everyone can, with time, become more mindful in life, even in the face of suffering. Focusing on the present moment – not thinking about the past and what has already happened, or the worrying about future and what has not yet happened (and might not ever happen) – is powerful. Historian Alice Morse Earle wrote: 'Every day may not be good, but there's something good in every day' – and, hey, that something good may just be a moment to be mindful.

Mindfulness does not have to be an exercise that you carve out 30 minutes for in your day (unless you would like to; apps such as Headspace or Calm have guided meditation – see Additional Resources, p. 263). Instead, it can easily be threaded into your day, every day. Weave consciousness into moments when you might otherwise go on autopilot; be mindful by intentionally bringing your mind and thoughts back to that moment. Appreciate the moment: how does it make you feel? Where are you? What is it about this moment that you would like to savour? Then remember to keep doing it and to keep practising it. Focus your attention completely on the moment, using some of the following techniques:

- **Taste:** the next time you eat or drink, without any external distractions, consciously absorb the aromas and flavours.

How does your food/drink taste? Notice the colour, texture and temperature. Become aware and appreciative of the food or drink you have in front of you – not everyone is fortunate enough to have it. Mindfully making and drinking a matcha is my favourite mindful moment (see p. 153).

- **Touch:** physical sensations could be anything from feeling the grass beneath your feet or the sand between your toes to the warmth of a log fire on the palms of your hands. Studies have shown that cuddling a pet, most likely your feline or canine companion, releases oxytocin in both human and pet, generating a calming and soothing effect.
- **Smell:** freshly cut grass, your mum's Sunday roast when it's almost ready to be served, the scent of your favourite perfume, the fresh smell of rain after a downpour . . . Or what about the pages of a brand-new book? Slowly breathe in, breathe out, and take a moment to feel the weight of the book in your hands, and the paper on your fingertips.
- **Sight:** wherever you are right now, look up. What can you see? Look again. What can you *really* see? Find something beautiful to appreciate. A delicate spider's web outside the window. Clouds rolling by. Ivy weaving its way up a wall.
- **Sound:** we are all bombarded with countless sounds daily but try to just focus on one. The hands of the clock ticking, or the sound of birds in the garden . . . If this does not work for you, try playing music (there is more on this to follow).

Mindful movement

It may also be possible to find mindfulness in movement. This could be when you are walking, cooking, cleaning, dancing, swimming or practising yoga. All of these activities can be experienced more consciously, but yoga is more specifically a mind-based therapy.

*

Adding mindfulness to your day does not seem so difficult now, I hope. But with life's many demands, perhaps it still seems impossible to you? Well, if the only time of the day you have to yourself is when you're taking a shower or brushing your teeth, could you try doing these things more mindfully? Take time to notice the smell of your shampoo, the heat of the water, the complete quiet and time for yourself . . .

The activities described below can also be exercised with awareness and intention. Mindfulness encourages a positive attitude, and pharmacist Raj comments that a positive mental attitude goes a long way to alleviating pain symptoms and cannot be underestimated. Not being defined by your condition and ensuring that you live life to the fullest, with whatever condition you may have is vital. In over 40 years, Raj has helped patients with all manner of conditions and those who are optimistic throughout exhibit markedly better outcomes and quality of life.

Stepping into nature

Growing up in a village on the edges of Yorkshire and Nottinghamshire, I was never far from nature, with long walks along the well-trodden tracks between farmers' fields. Even now, taking pathways in parks and woods, or by the river, alone or with a friend, with a book in tow or my music to listen to, is something that I love to do.

By the lake, by the trees or by the sea – wherever you find yourself in nature, it always feels good, doesn't it? But *why* and *how*? Japanese researchers in the 1980s provided the science to support what we instinctively know: that time spent immersed in nature is actually good for us. Termed '*shinrin-yoku*', which translates as 'forest bathing', it is a physiological and psychological 'ecotherapy' for the body.

But many cultures have long appreciated the importance of the natural world to human health for millennia. 'Biophilia', meaning the love of life and everything that is alive, hypothesises that humans have an 'innate tendency to focus on life and lifelike processes'. Being in nature is a guaranteed way to feel more connected, present and grateful. Good for our bodies and our brains, nature is proven to reduce heart rate, lower stress hormones, increase a sense of calm and relaxation, improve immune function, support breathing and counteract stress, anxiety and depression.

Considering that the human species has existed in modern surroundings for less than 0.01 per cent of our history, and the other 99.99 per cent living in nature, it should come as no surprise that we may yearn for and be drawn to natural environments. If you can step outside into nature once a day, or even immerse yourself in it for a whole day (sitting, lying, walking in it) – then do it; and do it mindfully, taking it in through all of your senses without any distractions. And for days when you are unable to step outside, bring a sample of nature inside instead: indoor foliage, houseplants and flowers do provide stress relief.

Creative crusade

Therapy of the creative or movement kind does not mean that you have to be the next Georgia O'Keeffe or Claude Monet, or as flexible as a yogi YouTuber. Being an expert is not required to feel the health benefits.

Written word

Taking the time (as you are now) to learn new information or to plunge your mind into an imagined world, simply by reading (for as little as six minutes) can reduce stress levels by 60 per cent, slowing your heartbeat, easing muscle tension and altering your state of mind. Writing and journaling ideas, feelings and events is therapeutic in a similar way. It does not matter if your writing is only legible to you – the act of being with your thoughts and writing them down has huge benefits for mental health. Writing in a stream-of-consciousness way, striking a conversation with yourself on the page, describing what is happening or has happened to you and how you are feeling, noting a list of things that you appreciate or are grateful for, logging your goals or achievements (big or small) finding space to express yourself freely and honestly – any or all of these may help you to process, de-stress and reset. Applying gratitude specifically through positive emotional writing has been shown to alleviate stress and anxiety.

Artistic licence

Whether it is doodling on some note paper, sketching a scene from your mind's eye or grabbing a paintbrush – the practice of art can be highly therapeutic. Here is your artistic licence to draw, scribble and splodge to your heart's content. *You go, Picasso*. Any form of art, no matter your experience (or lack of), has the capacity to reduce stress levels and provide emotional and motivational feelings of reward. And for patients with chronic illness, art has helped to improve overall health and wellbeing by distracting individuals from thoughts of illness, improving self-identity and providing a valuable social network.

There is also the enjoyment we feel at viewing artistic work, paintings and sculptures. Describe and ruminate on the art in front of you the next time you visit a gallery, museum or local art shop or fair. Or you could always buy art books packed with photographs of the real things. Beautiful artworks increase blood flow in a certain part of the brain inducing a 'feel-good' sensation – the equivalent of gazing at someone you love.

Medicinal music

Music, much like smell, sight and taste, has the power to take our minds back to old memories while simultaneously forming new ones. 'The piano keys are black and white, but they sound like a million colours in your mind.' I agree, Katie Melua. Being mindful when listening to music – thinking of how it makes you feel and the emotions it evokes – is a way to find inner calm. Whenever I am notified of a new album from an artist I like, I will take the time to lie in my bedroom or in the garden with my headphones on to really listen and take it in. Studies have shown a statistically significant reduction in depression levels over time with the use of music. A word of warning though: listening to your wedding song post-divorce may not have the same effect.

As well as listening to music, music therapy in the form of singing or playing has been reported to have a positive influence on anxiety and depression. Oh, and singing in the shower also counts!

Yoga: not just for the 'flexible'

Yoga is an ancient practice, over 2,000 years old. Praised for its broad-ranging benefits, both as a treatment and as a preventative form of healthcare, it has been shown to help increase flexibility, strength, mobility and balance, and may also reduce inflammation in the blood and reduce levels of cortisol (remember the stress hormone?), with tangible benefits for the whole body. It is a practice that can be gentle on the joints yet still be challenging for the body overall.

When yoga was suggested to me a few years ago, I snorted at the recommendation, but being on my yoga mat a few times or more a week, even if it is just for 15 minutes, really helps. Dr Lauren adds that the asanas (poses) in yoga encourage circulation of the synovial fluid of the joints, warming them up and promoting filtering out of the waste products of inflammation.

Initially, I tried doing a few yoga poses at home using YouTube videos, but struggled to know whether or not I was doing them properly. So, I would suggest trying a beginner's class in the types of yoga below, which are manageable and slower, and seeing how you get along. Yoga can be engaged with in a multitude of ways, from studios, gyms, outdoor or indoor yogi events, to online videos or channels. You can also fully immerse yourself by attending classes or retreats. It's multifaceted, and incorporates focused breathing, mental engagement, stress management, physical activity and mindfulness. It is an alternative to traditional exercise with potential psychological benefits and restorative effects. Putting any preconceived ideas aside, you may discover the benefits for yourself.

Chair-based yoga

This gentle form of yoga, as the name suggests, is practised sitting on a chair or using one for support during standing poses. It is ideal for chronic-pain conditions, if you have particularly limited mobility or if you want to practise yoga while at work.

Yin yoga – slow-paced yoga

The ultimate passive, calming and slow-paced yoga practice in which restorative poses are held for five minutes or more, this targets the deep connective tissues of the body, such as ligaments, joints and bones, rather than the muscles that are the focus of more physical practices, such as yang (opposite to yin). Highly meditative, it gives you the space to tune into both your mind and the physical sensations of your body. It may also be called restorative yoga, and props – including blocks, bolsters, blankets and straps – are used, so that you are supported in each of your poses comfortably.

For limited mobility, Viniyoga is adaptive and other styles that tend to be gentle include Anusara, Integral, Iyengar and Sivananda.

Breathwork and breathing techniques

As you read this, take a moment to pause and listen to your breathing. How is your body moving when you breathe? Try this:

- Place your left hand on your chest.
- Place your right hand on your abdomen.
- Breathe in and notice which hand moves first.

It is most likely to be your left hand, your shoulders rising as the air moves in and out at the top of your chest – this is shallow breathing that most of us tend to do daily. But ideally, you should feel your right hand move first, as your shoulders remain still and your tummy moves out:

- With your hands in the same position as above, relax and focus on inflating your belly.
- Bring in deep breaths.
- You should feel your right hand moving with your breaths.

Initially, it may feel strange or unnatural and it does require some practice. Check in with yourself in stressful moments (or any moments) and see if you have been unconsciously shallow breathing, then bring in the deep, mindful breathing from your belly instead. This form of yogic-controlled breathing reduces stress by slowing heart rate, dropping blood pressure and, in turn, helping us to feel relaxed. Use this form of breathing to do the following techniques:

Box breathing

Also known as square breathing, this is exactly what it says on the tin: there are four 'sides' to the technique and it is the perfect one to do before sleeping. If I'm struggling to sleep, it is my go-to technique. Either sitting or lying down, with your mouth closed, do the following:

- Breathe in for 4 seconds.
- Hold for 4 seconds.
- Breathe out for 4 seconds.

- Hold for 4 seconds.
- Repeat.

Ratio 2:1:2:1

Either sitting or lying down, start by doing this technique for 4 seconds, then work your way up to 6, 8, 10, over a period of time.

To start, 4:2:4:2 would be:

- Breathe in for 4 seconds
- Hold for 2 seconds
- Breathe out for 4 seconds
- Hold for 2 seconds

Now change the tempo by lengthening the time that you both hold your breath in and breathe out:

- 6 and 3 seconds: 6:3:6:3
- 8 and 4 seconds: 8:4:8:4

Setting Up Your Spaces

There is often a tendency for people to say that they are fine when, really, they are not. The Urban Dictionary jests that the phrase 'I'm fine' is the most-told lie in the English language (along with, 'I have read and agreed to the Terms and Conditions').

Perhaps rooted in this is the harmful societal expectation that someone who is struggling should simply 'get on with it' and 'not make a fuss', perpetuating the 'I'm fine' pretence and the stigma surrounding mental (especially) and physical health. In the USA, going to see a qualified therapist is as routine as going to the supermarket, but in the UK, therapy is seen as a huge step. Therapy is mind maintenance, just as dentistry is teeth maintenance. Not being able to communicate how you are truly feeling (to loved ones or a therapist) can have detrimental effects.

Communicating is easier said than done though. Speaking your truth takes the courage to be vulnerable and brave. To say, 'Hey, actually, I'm not fine. Can you help me?' can be the most difficult thing for a person to do. But downplaying how you are feeling and what you are going through can mean that you do not get the right support, the best treatment or the appropriate adjustments at work or at home.

As there are so many misconceptions surrounding arthritis in society, it can lead to people being dismissive of the condition or trivialising it. So those who are yet to be diagnosed or have already been diagnosed with arthritis may not feel comfortable enough to speak up, and as a result, feel disconnected and isolated, unable to access the help and support they need and deserve. It does not have to be this way.

Safe spaces

It is so vital to our wellbeing to have safe spaces, and in those spaces, to have safe people with whom we feel calm and comfortable enough with to talk about how we are feeling. In life, this may change over time and that is part of normal life.

Accepting when you need to rest, cooking for you, caring for you, FaceTiming or coming to you instead of asking you to leave the house – these are all forms of kindness the loved ones in your life might show or already be showing. Safe spaces include your own space, time, needs and boundaries. Setting your boundaries, being honest and true to yourself, is vital to maintaining a healthy mind, body and relationships. It can feel uncomfortable to say no to someone, but their reaction is not your responsibility, and if they love and respect you, they will respect your boundaries too.

Surround yourself with the right energy and the right people. Take a look and see who drags in toxicity, negativity, disrespect and contempt, and who brings joy, love, respect and kindness to you – then decide who you would most like to spend your time with. *Just a hint:* you deserve the latter (this extends to partners too). But sometimes the spaces that should be safe are not, or they do not provide you with what you need at the time when you need it.

For almost a year now, I have been going to therapy, and it has helped tremendously too. But acknowledging that not everyone has the privilege to afford going to therapy, it might be helpful to know that you can get a referral from your doctor, although waiting lists can be lengthy. Some therapists offer counselling on a sliding scale, where you pay a rate you can afford, while others offer free services. Some universities also provide it for free. Journaling, as already described, can help you to sort through your emotions, and, in addition, there is remote, text-based counselling via apps, as well as free helplines or face-to-face support individually and in groups run by charities.

Health spaces

We all expect our healthcare practitioners to be professional, compassionate, understanding and, well . . . patient with their patients. But they are only human. Maybe they are having a bad day, feeling tired or just not interpreting your needs properly (especially if you play down your symptoms). Either way, medical gaslighting (see p. 8) can make finding the right doctor or specialist taxing – a task made worse by the load laid on us by our arthritis and the urgency to find the right treatment.

Be prepared:

- In between appointments, write down how your arthritis has been, and how you have been physically feeling. Is the medication helping or not? Are diet and exercise making a difference? Capture anything you want to tell your doctor or rheumatologist and take these notes with you to your next appointment.
- Before appointments, read through what you have written above. What questions do you have for your healthcare professional? Take time to jot down any that you have.
- Record in photographic form improvements as well as any regression of your arthritis. It is helpful in tracking changes in your joints.

In the room:

- Be as direct and as informative as you can. It is hard not to be emotional at doctors' appointments, especially when you don't know what on earth is going on (pre-diagnosis), and I cannot count how many times I have been in tears. Breathe. Box breathe (see p. 249) if it helps. Say, 'Please give me one

moment. I am finding this difficult to talk about.' And try to compose yourself before continuing. It's okay to get upset, but know that with every appointment, you are hopefully getting closer to being able to manage your arthritis.
- Take notes during the consultation, especially if you are feeling particularly emotional; it will help you to remember and recall what was said. When my mum came to appointments, she would do this for me, so if you have someone you are able to bring in the room with you, that might help.
- Be honest – with yourself and with the doctor in front of you. You are both there for the same goal: to help you to feel and live better with your arthritis. If you are not being truthful or underplaying your symptoms, you probably will not receive the right treatment plan for your needs.
- Ask for a referral or go to alternative doctors or specialists if you feel that you are being medically gaslit, or know you are not getting the compassion and understanding that you deserve.

Work spaces

Work spaces can be difficult to navigate at the best of times, and it may be harder if your company has not employed someone with arthritis before.

Communicating with colleagues

There are a few things you may need to communicate with your work colleagues, such as time you might need for appointments, discussing a reduction in hours or working from home. It is essential that you do not allow anyone to make you feel guilty.

What is happening to you is out of your control and it is important that you emphasise this. Most people will surprise you and try to make things as comfortable for you as possible, as they will want the best for you and your health. If this is not the case, then get in touch with your HR representative to discuss any concerns you may have.

Adjustments for working well

Request ways that would make you more comfortable in your working day. This will vary from job to job – however, if your job is office based, speak to your company or HR representative about ergonomic equipment, including a chair, keyboard, mouse and desk. Do you have a long commuting day? If so, work from home when you need to. I had two laptops in one job, so that if I woke up in a flare, I could work from the comfort of my home (or bed). Working from home (if you can) is a viable, comfortable and economical way to work.

Know your rights. Typically, equal opportunity acts in various countries make it unlawful to discriminate against employees (including workers) because of a mental or physical disability.

Managing school and university

As you know, the bulk of my symptoms began at the start of my final year at university. This was terrifying to me, as someone who had never skipped a lecture and went to the library on weekends. I communicated with my lecturers and tutors about what I was going through, and adjustments were made: I was given extensions on essays, an online portal to access lectures and computer-based exams, as holding a pen was painful and difficult. If you are really struggling, apply to resit your exams if you are too poorly to attend due to arthritis. I missed a lot of lectures when I couldn't get out of bed – if they had been exams, I would have had to resit them.

Changing careers

This is a difficult one for me to write. Despite having bad days, I have been fortunate to have been given the support that I need and have been able to follow my passions. But for some, I know that this may not be the case. If you have had to change your career, is there something less strenuous but similar that you could try? If you have had to give up work entirely, is there something you enjoy doing? If so, could you start a blog or a YouTube channel about it? It may bring you joy and give you a purpose in the same way that your job did. It will be therapeutic too.

Online spaces

Online spaces can be good and bad, but you are the one in control. Would you have a certain person over for dinner? If the answer is no, then why are you looking at their social-media content every day, especially when it makes you feel rubbish? You choose who you invite into your home and physical world, so be just as selective with who you invite into your digital world. And choose wisely.

I have started using app time limits (Settings —> Screen Time —> App Limits), available on most mainstream smartphones, to reduce my digital and social-media consumption. The news and media can be anxiety-inducing, as can somebody's social-media highlight reel. There are numerous Photoshopping-detox-tea-drinking dipsticks out there, and they are *not* soul-nourishing.

An old parable goes that we have two fighting wolves within us: one is evil – angry, greedy, jealous, arrogant and cowardly; the other is good – peaceful, loving, modest, generous, honest and trustworthy. The one that wins, is the one you feed. Take a look at your social-media wolves, make an assessment and click 'mute', 'unfollow' or 'block' where required. Ultimately, comparison is the thief of joy, as I said before. And it is futile, because only *you* define *you* and who you are, and there is just one of you. Isn't that a gift? I think it is. I know it is. *Start telling yourself that it is.*

Support without the face-to-face

- Facebook groups
- Social-media pages
- Blogs and websites

You may find support in these places and discover someone or something that you can relate to. But be careful and remember those wolves: some support groups are scaremongering and upsetting; others are more uplifting, and they are the ones I would recommend. You can get a sense of an online community when you step inside it – if it does not feel right or provide any nourishment to your good wolf, then politely leave.

Use your voice and share your story

- Charity-sponsored activities
- Contributing to online forums and communities
- Volunteering to guest-write for arthritis charities
- Signing petitions, speaking to your local government

Never underestimate the power of your story, your courage and setbacks, your successes and joys and everything in between – how your story has the ability to help someone else feel they are being seen; someone who may have struggled without it. If you are able to share your story, you can do so in varying ways. Perhaps you could raise money for an arthritis research charity, provide answers to questions asked in online forums or Facebook groups, contribute to blogs about your condition or sign petitions to better care for people living with arthritis. It should feel cathartic and therapeutic; helping others may, in turn, help you to feel better. It's a lovely cycle to be in.

If I had not shared my story, I might still be struggling, feeling isolated and alone. I will never forget the day Eva's father reached out to me on Instagram. Eva is 10 years old and was diagnosed with juvenile arthritis when she was just 3 years old. According to her dad, she loves watching my Instagram stories: 'I think you are super cool!!' she wrote to me. 'You inspire me to do great things and eat healthier, thanks a lot!!'

Even if you help just one person in the world besides yourself, this means that you and this person have benefited from the arthritis you are both afflicted with, and you both feel happier in knowing you are not the only one.

A Final Word

So, you may ask: will this book help me to manage my arthritis or AID?

And the answer? This book is a guide, and truthfully it is up to you how much or how little you implement into your daily life. There is a whole mixture of things that may alleviate or worsen your symptoms – because each person will experience their condition differently. The book is by no means a replacement for your current therapy or medication, but an addition to it. Do not be disheartened if you are unable to do all of it at once; do what you can when you can, and enjoy each step as you go, knowing that you are taking care of you.

Dr Jenna Macciochi writes:

> 'There is no denying the challenges of battling a chronic illness like RA. But it is also an opportunity to seize the reins and take proactive steps to strike a balanced lifestyle. With the right choices, like a Mediterranean-focused diet and stress management, you will be able to regain a sense of agency over your health which is of great psychological – and therefore immunological – importance and can play a huge role in how you feel, cope and manage your condition.'

Victoria Jain adds, 'In most cases, improving nutrition can help to reduce symptoms of AID, and even put the condition into remission. With a healthy anti-inflammatory diet, full of nourishing nutrient-dense foods, you give your body the best chance to heal and function properly again.'

We must all find the time to appreciate and be thankful for our lives, our bodies and the greater world around us. In the words of Oprah Winfrey: 'As long as you are breathing, there is more right with you than wrong with you, no matter what is wrong.' Accepting the things we have and cannot change, with the courage to change the ones that we can may give us a different perspective. You have shown courage already – just by reading this book, you are beginning to accept that you live with arthritis and have the bravery to embark on making changes to your life for the better. Changes that are in your control, whether that is the food and drink you consume, the exercise you do, the pain relief you try, the way you view your arthritis and the people you spend your time with – on- or offline. All of these are within your power, and so are the tools to help you live well *and live better* with arthritis – and beat it naturally.

Worth a Read

There are a number of authors, from recipe writers to academics and health practitioners, to whom I am indebted. Some I discovered when I had almost completed my manuscript (with new and enlightening research that I had to scramble in), while others inspired me from the very beginning – and a few I have been grateful to have met. If you have enjoyed the content of this book and would like to explore further and expand your knowledge in any number of subject areas, please refer to the list of select (wonderful) humans below.

In alphabetical order:

- Scott C. Anderson with John F. Cryan and Ted Dinan, *The Psychobiotic Revolution: Mood, Food, and the New Science of the Gut-Brain Connection*
- Dr Rupy Aujla – *The Doctor's Kitchen: Eat to beat illness*
- Edward Bullmore – *The Inflamed Mind: A radical new approach to depression*
- Patrizia Collard – *The Little Book of Mindfulness: 10 Minutes a Day to Less Stress, More Peace*
- Giulia Enders – *GUT: the inside story of our body's most underrated organ*
- Dr Dani Gordan – *The CBD Bible: Cannabis and the Wellness Revolution That Will Change Your Life*
- Michael Greger – *How Not to Die: Discover the Foods*

Scientifically Proven to Prevent and Reverse Disease

- Dr Jenna Macciochi – *Immunity: the Science of Staying Well*
- Dr Michael Mosley – *The Clever Guts Diet*
- Nick Potter – *The Meaning of Pain: What it is, why we feel it, and how to overcome it*
- Andy Puddicombe – *The Headspace Guide to Meditation and Mindfulness*
- Dr Megan Rossi – *Eat Yourself Healthy*
- Tim Spector – *The Diet Myth: The Real Science Behind What We Eat*
- Matthew Walker – *Why We Sleep*

Additional Resources

Mindfulness Support Via Apps

- HeadSpace
- Calm

Nutritional Tracking Via Apps

- MyFitnessPal – tracks nutrients and vitamins of foods

Counselling Via Apps

- Babylon
- PlusGuidance
- BetterHelp
- Talkspace

Charities

There are also free helplines and face-to-face support, both individually and in groups run by charities; these may vary depending on your location, but the main UK and US ones are as follows:

In the UK

Samaritans UK

For confidential, non-judgemental emotional support.

116 123 (24 hours a day, free to call)

Mind UK

For information and support with mental health.

0300 123 3393 (9am-6pm Monday to Friday) or text 86463

The Mix UK

Support service for 13–25-year-olds.

0808 808 4994 (11am–11pm, free to call) or text 'THEMIX' to 85258

Versus Arthritis

0800 5200 520 for free (Monday–Friday, 9am–8pm)

NRAS (National Rheumatoid Arthritis Society)

0800 298 7650 (Monday–Friday, 9.30am–4.30pm, free from landlines or ask for a call back)

In the USA

Samaritans USA

(877) 870-4673 (24 hours a day, 7 days a week, free to call and text)

Mental Health America

1-800-273-8255 or text MHA to 741741 (24 hours, 7 days a week, free to call and text).

SAMHSA (US Government Health Body)

1-800-985-5990 (24 hours a day, 7 days a week, free to call)

Arthritis Foundation USA

1-800-283-7800 (free to call)

Additional arthritis charities

- Arthritis Action – UK
- Psoriasis Association – UK

- Arthritis Ireland – Ireland
- Arthritis National Research Foundation – USA
- National Psoriasis Foundation – USA
- Arthritis Society – Canada
- Arthritis Australia – Australia
- The Rheumatism Line (Reumatiker Linjen) – Sweden
- AFPric Association de Patients – France
- The National Association of Patients with Childhood Arthritis and Rheumatisms (A Associação Nacional de Doentes com Artrites e Reumatismos da Infância (A.N.D.A.I.) – Portugal
- National Arthritis Coordinating Association (Asociación Coordinadora Nacional de Artritis) – Spain
- The German Rheumatism League (Die Deutsche Rheuma-Liga) – Germany
- ANMAR Onlus National Association of Rheumatic Diseases (ANMAR Onlus Associazione Nazionale Malattie Reumatiche) – Italy

Acknowledgements

To my mum, Rachael, and my sister, Katy – there are no words to truly explain how thankful and grateful I am for your love and endless support. Mum, you phenomenally and gracefully have carried the weight of being two parents. I am indebted to you and your devotion to us both. You gave us the life Dad had imagined for us. Thank you for your strength, guidance and love – for everything. My little sister, Katy: thank you for always being there for me, from the trivial to the tough times. For keeping me grounded and embracing my weird and whimsical spirit since you came into the world.

And to another heroine: my Grandma Anne. Tenaciously honest and unwaveringly independent. You are more than a grandparent; you are a dear friend and I treasure your friendship. Thank you for your ferocious energy, enthusiasm and advocacy during my whole life.

To Mahi Iftikhar, I am so thankful for our friendship. Your generous support, excitement and honest advice (including recipe tasting) for Arthritis Foodie has been invaluable, and I appreciate you so very much. Thank you for believing in me, inspiring me and being there for me on good days and difficult days too.

A huge thank you to my team at Yellow Kite Books, copy editor Anne Newman, assistant editor Holly Whitaker, and especially to my editor and publisher Carolyn Thorne for seeing the potential of this book and shaping it into what it has become. You have helped me to create the book that I envisaged, and more.

Many thanks to Lee Constantine, at Publishizer, for believing in the concept and idea of this book before I had even put pen to paper. And to Jackie, who introduced me to Lee and the publishing world that felt very obscure and unattainable to me at the time. I must add a thank you here to Rachel Hall too, who proudly revealed my idea for the book to Jackie, and who is a constant source of support. Gratitude to Dr Rupy Aujla too, who warmly listened to my idea for this book and encouraged me to pursue it.

To my brilliant contributors, as listed in the beginning, for big-heartedly and kindly giving up their time to provide insightful and important information that will help the lives of so many people living with arthritis. Thank you for endorsing and adding no end of value to this book. I am so grateful. And my thanks also to the many researchers globally who work to bring to light exciting new insights into medicine, nutrition, and health.

To my close friends and family, who continuously provide so much love and reassurance - thank you for championing everything that I have dreamed of doing: Evangalene Mcleod, Laura Whitehouse, Jack Roberts, Dayana Calambas Collazos, Azera Jones, Charlotte Flach, Sarah Stephenson, Gemma Senior, Priyanka Nehra, Shyam Janani, Emma Middleton, Izzie Wood and Tasha Wood. And to my lovely stepdad Stephen Wood for his patience, kindness and generosity. A special mention to Rebecca Crawforth, for encouraging my dreams since we met and for being an astounding role model. A word of thanks to the Johnsons too: Grandpa, Bethany, Andrew, William, and Russell. I cherish all of you, and many more wonderful friends and extended family it would take too long to name – I will make sure that you know who you are.

An enormous thank you to anyone who has been a part of the Arthritis Foodie community from day one to the days that have followed since. I am eternally grateful for your support, encouragement, and comfort. You have granted me the platform to bring this important message to the world. Particular appreciation goes to those of you who believed in this book before you could hold it in your hands, and pre-ordered in 2019. There are too many of you to name but thank you to those who have invested substantially and have not already been mentioned: Michael Speight, Sharm Vara, Liv Gray, Kirsty Brown, Paul Fishpool, Ioana Mistreanu, Kara McInnis, Sally Wren, Steph Burt, Belinda Hardman, Ben Ho, Helen Mortimer, Kate Porter, Nicola Cromwell-Redford, Sally Wren, Shelley Hayward and Yvonne Jacobs.

Finally, though you cannot read this, to Dad, for imparting the confidence and the courage in me to fearlessly 'knock on doors' of opportunity, accepting that the worst thing that can happen is the door not opening. I miss your big heart every day.

References

Introduction

1. Pahwa R, Goyal A, Bansal P, et al. 'Chronic Inflammation' (2020). In:Treasure Island (FL): StatPearls Publishing. Retrieved from: https://www.ncbi.nlm.nih.gov/books/NBK493173/.
2. Versus Arthritis (2019). 'The State of Musculoskeletal Health 2019.' *versusarthritis.org*. Retrieved from: https://www.versusarthritis.org/media/14594/state-of-musculoskeletal-health-2019.pdf.

Chapter 1

1. Global Burden of Disease Study 2013 Collaborators (2015). Global, regional, and national incidence, prevalence, and years lived with disability for 301 acute and chronic diseases and injuries in 188 countries, 1990-2013: a systematic analysis for the Global Burden of Disease Study 2013. *Lancet (London, England)*, *386*(9995), 743–800. https://doi.org/10.1016/S0140-6736(15)60692-4.
2. Watanabe. K, *et al.* (2014). 'Chapter 12 - Kampo Medicines for Autoimmune Disorders: Rheumatoid Arthritis and Autoimmune Diabetes Mellitus' in Japanese Kampo Medicines for the Treatment of Common Diseases: Focus on Inflammation, *Academic Press, 2017*, pp. 103-110, https://doi.org/10.1016/B978-0-12-809398-6.00012-3.
3. Vojdani, A., Pollard, K. M., & Campbell, A. W. (2014). Environmental triggers and autoimmunity. *Autoimmune diseases*, *2014*, 798029. https://doi.org/10.1155/2014/798029.
4. Dragos, D., Gilca, M., Gaman, L., Vlad, A., Iosif, L., Stoian, I., & Lupescu, O. (2017). Phytomedicine in Joint Disorders. *Nutrients*, *9(1)*, 70. doi:10.3390/nu9010070.
5. Houard, X., Goldring, M. B., & Berenbaum, F. (2013). Homeostatic mechanisms in articular cartilage and role of inflammation in osteoarthritis. *Current rheumatology reports*, *15*(11), 375. https://doi.org/10.1007/s11926-013-0375-6.

6. Zhang, J. M., & An, J. (2007). Cytokines, inflammation, and pain. *International anesthesiology clinics*, *45*(2), 27–37. https://doi.org/10.1097/AIA.0b013e318034194e.
7. O'Shea J.J, Gadina M., Siegel, R.M. (2019). 9 - Cytokines and Cytokine Receptors, *Clinical Immunology (Fifth Edition), 127-155.e1*, https://doi.org/10.1016/B978-0-7020-6896-6.00009-0.
8. Yang, C. L., Or, T. C., Ho, M. H., & Lau, A. S. (2013). Scientific basis of botanical medicine as alternative remedies for rheumatoid arthritis. *Clinical reviews in allergy & immunology*, *44*(3), 284–300. https://doi.org/10.1007/s12016-012-8329-8.
9. Ismail, Samir. (2013). 'Anti-Inflammatory and Anti-Arthritic Activity of Some Spices Extracts on Adjuvant Induced Arthritis in Rats', *Journal of Applied Sciences Research 2013*, *9*(8):5303-531.
10. Cojocaru, M., Cojocaru, I. M., Silosi, I., Vrabie, C. D., & Tanasescu, R. (2010). Extra-articular Manifestations in Rheumatoid Arthritis. *Maedica*, *5*(4), 286–291. Retrieved from: https://www.ncbi.nlm.nih.gov/pmc/articles/PMC3152850/.
11. Alunno, A., Carubbi, F., Giacomelli, R., & Gerli, R. (2017). Cytokines in the pathogenesis of rheumatoid arthritis: new players and therapeutic targets. *BMC rheumatology*, *1*, 3. https://doi.org/10.1186/s41927-017-0001-8.
12. Mahajna, H., Mahroum, N., & Amital, H. (2015). 'Rheumatoid Arthritis and Infections: More Than an Association?', In Yehuda Shoenfeld, Nancy Agmon-Levin, Noel R. Rose (Eds), *Infection and Autoimmunity (Second Edition), Academic Press, 2015*, pp. 729-734, https://doi.org/10.1016/B978-0-444-63269-2.00065-9.
13. Chirali I.Z. (2014). Cupping Therapy Evidence-Based Research. *Traditional Chinese Medicine Cupping Therapy (Third Edition)*, pp. 247-310, https://doi.org/10.1016/B978-0-7020-4352-9.00016-3.
14. Wright.V, Moll J.M.H (1976). Psoriatic arthritis. Seronegative polyarthritis. *Seminars in Arthritis and Rheumatism,* 3(1), pp. 169–223. https://doi.org/10.1016/0049-0172(73)90035-8.
15. O'Rielly, D. D., & Rahman, P. (2014). Genetics of psoriatic arthritis. *Best practice & research. Clinical rheumatology*, *28*(5), 673–685. https://doi.org/10.1016/j.berh.2014.10.010.
16. Gladman, D. D., Antoni, C., Mease, P., Clegg, D. O., & Nash, P. (2005). Psoriatic arthritis: epidemiology, clinical features, course, and outcome. *Annals of the rheumatic diseases*, *64 Suppl 2*(Suppl 2), ii14–ii17. https://doi.org/10.1136/ard.2004.032482
17. Kane. D (2015), 42 - Musculoskeletal ultrasound, *Rheumatology (Sixth Edition),* 1(42) pp. 331-341, https://doi.org/10.1016/

B978-0-323-09138-1.00042-5. Retrieved from: https://www.sciencedirect.com/science/article/pii/B9780323091381000425.

18. Gottlieb, A., & Merola, J. F. (2019). Psoriatic arthritis for dermatologists. *The Journal of dermatological treatment*, 1–18. Advance online publication. https://doi.org/10.1080/09546634.2019.1605142.
19. NHS England UK (2018, December, 14). Overview of Arthritis. *NHS England UK*. Retrieved April, 11, 2020 from: https://www.nhs.uk/conditions/arthritis/.
20. Nordal E, Rygg M, Fasth A (2015). 101 - Clinical features of juvenile idiopathic arthritis, *Rheumatology (Sixth Edition)*, 1(101), pp. 833-844, https://doi.org/10.1016/B978-0-323-09138-1.00101-7.
21. Malattia C, Martini A (2020), Chapter 35 - Juvenile Idiopathic Arthritis, *The Autoimmune Diseases (Sixth Edition), Academic Press*, pp. 675-690, https://doi.org/10.1016/B978-0-12-812102-3.00035-X.
22. Foster, H. E., Marshall, N., Myers, A., Dunkley, P., & Griffiths, I. D. (2003). Outcome in adults with juvenile idiopathic arthritis: a quality of life study. *Arthritis and rheumatism*, *48*(3), 767–775. https://doi.org/10.1002/art.10863.
23. Hong D.K., Gutierrez K (2018), 77 - Infectious and Inflammatory Arthritis, *Principles and Practice of Pediatric Infectious Diseases (Fifth Edition)*, Elsevier, pp. 487-493.e3, https://doi.org/10.1016/B978-0-323-40181-4.00077-3.
24. Berbari E.F, Osmon D.R, Steckelberg J. M. (2010), Chapter 40 - Infective and reactive arthritis, *Infectious Diseases (Third Edition)*, pp. 438-444, https://doi.org/10.1016/B978-0-323-04579-7.00040-X.
25. Burgos-Vargas R, Vázquez-Mellado J (2011), Chapter 39 - REACTIVE ARTHRITIS, *Textbook of Pediatric Rheumatology (Sixth Edition)*, pp. 591-599, https://doi.org/10.1016/B978-1-4160-6581-4.10039-1.
26. Gutierrez K (2012), 79 - Infectious and Inflammatory Arthritis, *Principles and Practice of Pediatric Infectious Diseases (Fourth Edition)*, pp. 477-483.e4, https://doi.org/10.1016/B978-1-4377-2702-9.00079-9.
27. Versus Arthritis (2013, November). Reactive Arthritis. *Arthritis Research UK*. Retrieved April, 11, 2020 from: https://www.versusarthritis.org/media/1324/reactive-arthritis-information-booklet.pdf.
28. Rowdon G e.t al (2008), Chapter 10 - Arthritic, Metabolic, and Vascular Disorders, *Baxter's the Foot and Ankle in Sport (Second Edition)*, pp. 241-249, https://doi.org/10.1016/B978-032302358-0.10010-7.
29. McLean L, 187 - Etiology and pathogenesis of gout, *Rheumatology (Sixth Edition)*, pp. 1555-1568, https://doi.org/10.1016/B978-0-323-09138-1.00187-X.
30. Wolff D (2007), Gout, *The Comprehensive Pharmacology*, pp. 1-8, https://doi.org/10.1016/B978-008055232-3.60681-6.

31. Pande I (2006), An update on gout, *Indian Journal of Rheumatology*, 1(2), pp. 60-65, https://doi.org/10.1016/S0973-3698(10)60005-2.
32. Brower A C, Flemming D J (2012),16 - Gout, *Arthritis in Black and White (Third Edition)*, pp. 293-308, https://doi.org/10.1016/B978-1-4160-5595-2.00016-X.
33. Hameed F A (2018), Chapter 69 - Gout, *Integrative Medicine (Fourth Edition)*, pp. 689-696.e2, https://doi.org/10.1016/B978-0-323-35868-2.00069-4.
34. Pizzorno J E et al (2016), 31 - Gout, *The Clinician's Handbook of Natural Medicine (Third Edition)*, pp. 347-354, https://doi.org/10.1016/B978-0-7020-5514-0.00040-3.
35. Cotán D et al (2014). Chapter 10 - Mitophagy Plays a Protective Role in Fibroblasts from Patients with Coenzyme Q10 Deficiency, *Autophagy: Cancer, Other Pathologies, Inflammation, Immunity, Infection, and Aging, Academic Press*, pp. 131-144, https://doi.org/10.1016/B978-0-12-405530-8.00010-8.
36. Sancassiani, F., Machado, S., Ruggiero, V., Cacace, E., Carmassi, C., Gesi, C., Dell'Osso, L., & Carta, M. G. (2017). The management of fibromyalgia from a psychosomatic perspective: an overview. *International review of psychiatry (Abingdon, England)*, *29*(5), 473–488. https://doi.org/10.1080/09540261.2017.1320982.
37. de Heer, E. W., Vriezekolk, J. E., & van der Feltz-Cornelis, C. M. (2017). Poor Illness Perceptions Are a Risk Factor for Depressive and Anxious Symptomatology in Fibromyalgia Syndrome: A Longitudinal Cohort Study. *Frontiers in psychiatry*, *8*, 217. https://doi.org/10.3389/fpsyt.2017.00217.
38. Mendelson S.D (2008), 4 - METABOLIC SYNDROME AND PSYCHIATRIC ILLNESS, *Metabolic Syndrome and Psychiatric Illness*, pp. 49-72, https://doi.org/10.1016/B978-012374240-7.50006-1.
39. Niesters M, Dahan A (2017), Fibromyalgia, *Reference Module in Neuroscience and Biobehavioral Psychology*, https://doi.org/10.1016/B978-0-12-809324-5.04240-1.
40. Aranow C, et.al (2019), 51 - Systemic Lupus Erythematosus, *Clinical Immunology (Fifth Edition)*, pp. 685-704.e1, https://doi.org/10.1016/B978-0-7020-6896-6.00051-X.
41. Hauser R A (2010), The acceleration of articular cartilage degeneration in osteoarthritis by nonsteroidal anti-inflammatory drugs, *Journal of Prolotherapy*, pp 305-322. Retrieved from: http://journalofprolotherapy.com/the-acceleration-of-articular-cartilage-degeneration-in-osteoarthritis-by-nonsteroidal-anti-inflammatory-drugs/.
42. Mackesy C. (2019). *The Boy, the Mole, the Fox and the Horse*, London: Ebury Publishing.

43. Vighi, G., Marcucci, F., Sensi, L., Di Cara, G., & Frati, F. (2008). Allergy and the gastrointestinal system. *Clinical and experimental immunology*, 153 Suppl 1(Suppl 1), 3–6. https://doi.org/10.1111/j.1365-2249.2008.03713.x.
44. Mosley M. (2017), *The Clever Guts Diet: How to Revolutionise Your Body from the Inside Out,* London: Short Books.
45. Codella, R., Luzi, L., & Terruzzi, I. (2018). Exercise has the guts: How physical activity may positively modulate gut microbiota in chronic and immune-based diseases. *Digestive and liver disease: official journal of the Italian Society of Gastroenterology and the Italian Association for the Study of the Liver*, *50*(4), 331–341. https://doi.org/10.1016/j.dld.2017.11.016.
46. Sender, R., Fuchs, S., & Milo, R. (2016). Revised Estimates for the Number of Human and Bacteria Cells in the Body. *PLoS biology*, *14*(8), e1002533. https://doi.org/10.1371/journal.pbio.1002533.
47. Anderson S C, Cryan J F, Dinan T. (2017). *The Psychobiotic Revolution: Mood, Food, and the New Science of the Gut-Brain Connection,* Washington DC: National Geographic.
48. Macchiochi J (2020), *Immunity: The Science of Staying Well,* London: Thorsons.
49. Mosley M. (2017), *The Clever Guts Diet: How to Revolutionise Your Body from the Inside Out,* London: Short Books.
50. Anderson S C, Cryan J F, Dinan T. (2017). *The Psychobiotic Revolution: Mood, Food, and the New Science of the Gut-Brain Connection,* Washington DC: National Geographic.
51. Macaninch E, Buckner L, Amin P, et al (2020), Time for nutrition in medical education, *BMJ Nutrition, Prevention & Health*. doi: 10.1136/bmjnph-2019-000049.
52. Carrera-Quintanar, L., López Roa, R. I., Quintero-Fabián, S., Sánchez-Sánchez, M. A., Vizmanos, B., & Ortuño-Sahagún, D. (2018). Phytochemicals That Influence Gut Microbiota as Prophylactics and for the Treatment of Obesity and Inflammatory Diseases. *Mediators of inflammation*. https://doi.org/10.1155/2018/9734845.
53. Kau, A. L., Ahern, P. P., Griffin, N. W., Goodman, A. L., & Gordon, J. I. (2011). Human nutrition, the gut microbiome and the immune system. *Nature*, *474*(7351), pp. 327–336. https://doi.org/10.1038/nature10213.
54. Forbes JD, Van Domselaar G and Bernstein CN (2016) The Gut Microbiota in Immune-Mediated Inflammatory Diseases. Front. Microbiol. 7:1081. doi: 10.3389/fmicb.2016.01081 https://www.frontiersin.org/articles/10.3389/fmicb.2016.01081/full.
55. Bach-Faig, A., Berry, E. M., Lairon, D., Reguant, J., Trichopoulou, A., Dernini, S., Medina, F. X., Battino, M., Belahsen, R., Miranda, G., Serra-Majem, L.,

& Mediterranean Diet Foundation Expert Group (2011). Mediterranean diet pyramid today. Science and cultural updates. *Public health nutrition*, *14*(12A), 2274–2284. https://doi.org/10.1017/S1368980011002515.

56. Khanna, S., Jaiswal, K. S., & Gupta, B. (2017). Managing Rheumatoid Arthritis with Dietary Interventions. *Frontiers in nutrition*, *4*, 52. https://doi.org/10.3389/fnut.2017.00052.
57. Tomasello, G., Mazzola, M., Leone, A., Sinagra, E., Zummo, G., Farina, F., Damiani, P., Cappello, F., Gerges Geagea, A., Jurjus, A., Bou Assi, T., Messina, M., & Carini, F. (2016). Nutrition, oxidative stress and intestinal dysbiosis: Influence of diet on gut microbiota in inflammatory bowel diseases. *Biomedical papers of the Medical Faculty of the University Palacky, Olomouc, Czechoslovakia*, *160*(4), 461–466. https://doi.org/10.5507/bp.2016.052.
58. Casas, R., Sacanella, E., Urpí-Sardà, M., Corella, D., Castañer, O., Lamuela-Raventos, R. M., Salas-Salvadó, J., Martínez-González, M. A., Ros, E., & Estruch, R. (2016). Long-Term Immunomodulatory Effects of a Mediterranean Diet in Adults at High Risk of Cardiovascular Disease in the PREvención con DIeta MEDiterránea (PREDIMED) Randomized Controlled Trial. *The Journal of nutrition*, *146*(9), 1684–1693. https://doi.org/10.3945/jn.115.229476.
59. Santangelo, C., Vari, R., Scazzocchio, B., De Sanctis, P., Giovannini, C., D'Archivio, M., & Masella, R. (2018). Anti-inflammatory Activity of Extra Virgin Olive Oil Polyphenols: Which Role in the Prevention and Treatment of Immune-Mediated Inflammatory Diseases?. *Endocrine, metabolic & immune disorders drug targets*, *18*(1), 36–50. https://doi.org/10.2174/1871530317666171114114321.
60. Pearson, C. M., Wood, F. D., Mcdaniel, E. G., & DAFT, F. S. (1963). Adjuvant arthritis induced in germ-free rats. *Proceedings of the Society for Experimental Biology and Medicine. Society for Experimental Biology and Medicine (New York, N.Y.)*, *112*, 91–93. https://doi.org/10.3181/00379727-112-27959.
61. Kohashi, O., Kuwata, J., Umehara, K., Uemura, F., Takahashi, T., & Ozawa, A. (1979). Susceptibility to adjuvant-induced arthritis among germfree, specific-pathogen-free, and conventional rats. *Infection and immunity*, *26*(3), 791–794. https://doi.org/10.1128/IAI.26.3.791-794.1979.
62. Kohashi, O., Kohashi, Y., Takahashi, T., Ozawa, A., & Shigematsu, N. (1985). Reverse effect of gram-positive bacteria vs. gram-negative bacteria on adjuvant-induced arthritis in germfree rats. *Microbiology and immunology*, *29*(6), 487–497. https://doi.org/10.1111/j.1348-0421.1985.tb00851.x.
63. Versus Arthritis (2020, June), Does gut Bacteria Play a Role in Rheumatoid Arthritis?. *Versus Arthritis*. Retrieved June, 26, 2020 from: https://www.

versusarthritis.org/news/2020/june/does-gut-bacteria-play-a-role-in-rheumatoid-arthritis/.

64. Liu, X., Zeng, B., Zhang, J., Li, W., Mou, F., Wang, H., Zou, Q., Zhong, B., Wu, L., Wei, H., & Fang, Y. (2016). Role of the Gut Microbiome in Modulating Arthritis Progression in Mice. *Scientific reports*, 6, 30594. https://doi.org/10.1038/srep30594.
65. Zhang, X., Zhang, D., et al, (2015). The oral and gut microbiomes are perturbed in rheumatoid arthritis and partly normalized after treatment. *Nature medicine*, 21(8), 895–905. https://doi.org/10.1038/nm.3914.
66. Scher, J. U., Sczesnak, A., Longman, R. S., Segata, N., Ubeda, C., Bielski, C., Rostron, T., Cerundolo, V., Pamer, E. G., Abramson, S. B., Huttenhower, C., & Littman, D. R. (2013). Expansion of intestinal *Prevotella copri* correlates with enhanced susceptibility to arthritis. *eLife*, 2, e01202. https://doi.org/10.7554/eLife.01202.
67. Maeda, Y., et al, (2016). Dysbiosis Contributes to Arthritis Development via Activation of Autoreactive T Cells in the Intestine. *Arthritis & rheumatology (Hoboken, N.J.)*, 68(11), 2646–2661. https://doi.org/10.1002/art.39783.
68. Eerola, E., Möttönen, T., Hannonen, P., Luukkainen, R., Kantola, I., Vuori, K., Tuominen, J., & Toivanen, P. (1994). Intestinal flora in early rheumatoid arthritis. *British journal of rheumatology, 33(11)*, 1030–1038. https://doi.org/10.1093/rheumatology/33.11.1030.
69. Jethwa, H., & Abraham, S. (2017). The evidence for microbiome manipulation in inflammatory arthritis. *Rheumatology (Oxford, England)*, *56*(9), 1452–1460. https://doi.org/10.1093/rheumatology/kew374.
70. Scher, J. U., Sczesnak, A., Longman, R. S., Segata, N., Ubeda, C., Bielski, C., Rostron, T., Cerundolo, V., Pamer, E. G., Abramson, S. B., Huttenhower, C., & Littman, D. R. (2013). Expansion of intestinal *Prevotella copri* correlates with enhanced susceptibility to arthritis. *eLife*, 2, e01202. https://doi.org/10.7554/eLife.01202.
71. Badsha H. (2018). Role of Diet in Influencing Rheumatoid Arthritis Disease Activity. *The open rheumatology journal*, *12*, 19–28. https://doi.org/10.2174/1874312901812010019.

References – Chapter 2

1. Hekmatpou, D., Mehrabi, F., Rahzani, K., & Aminiyan, A. (2019). The Effect of Aloe Vera Clinical Trials on Prevention and Healing of Skin Wound: A Systematic Review. *Iranian journal of medical sciences*, *44*(1), 1–9. https://www.ncbi.nlm.nih.gov/pmc/articles/PMC6330525/.

2. Bassett, I.B., Barnetson, R.S.C. and Pannowitz, D.L. (1990). A comparative study of tea-tree oil versus benzoylperoxide in the treatment of acne. *Medical Journal of Australia*, 153: 455-458. doi:10.5694/j.1326-5377.1990.tb126150.x.
3. Halstead, F. D., Rauf, M., Moiemen, N. S., Bamford, A., Wearn, C. M., Fraise, A. P., Lund, P. A., Oppenheim, B. A., & Webber, M. A. (2015). The Antibacterial Activity of Acetic Acid against Biofilm-Producing Pathogens of Relevance to Burns Patients. *PloS one*, *10*(9), e0136190. https://doi.org/10.1371/journal.pone.0136190.
4. World Health Organisation. (2002). Traditional Medicine Strategy Launched, *WHO News, Geneva, Switzerland,* vol. 80 of 610.
5. Ahmad, Iqbal & Zahin, Maryam & Aqil, Farrukh & Hasan, Sameena & Khan, Mohd & Owais, Mohd. (2008). Bioactive compounds from *Punica granatum*, *Curcuma longa* and *Zingiber officinale* and their therapeutic potential. *Drugs of The Future - DRUG FUTURE. 33.* 10.1358/dof.2008.033.04.1186159.
6. Seward, E.A., Kelly, S. (2016). Dietary nitrogen alters codon bias and genome composition in parasitic microorganisms. *Genome Biol 17, 22.* https://doi.org/10.1186/s13059-016-1087-9.
7. Woolston C. (2020). White men still dominate in UK academic science. *Nature, 579(7800),* 622. https://doi.org/10.1038/d41586-020-00759-1.
8. Dragos, D., Gilca, M., Gaman, L., Vlad, A., Iosif, L., Stoian, I., & Lupescu, O. (2017). Phytomedicine in Joint Disorders. *Nutrients*, *9*(1), 70. https://doi.org/10.3390/nu9010070.
9. Dr Rupy Aujla. (14th April 2020). 'The Role of Food in Health', *TEDxBristol*. Retrieved from https://www.youtube.com/watch?v=yTQ0tBmLbns.
10. Nahar L., Xiao J., Sarker S.D (2020). Introduction of Phytonutrients. In: Xiao J., Sarker S., Asakawa Y. (eds) *Handbook of Dietary Phytochemicals*. Springer, Singapore. https://doi.org/10.1007/978-981-13-1745-3_2-1.
11. Gupta, Charu, and Dhan Prakash. 'Phytonutrients as therapeutic agents'. Journal of Complementary and Integrative Medicine 11.3: 151-169. https://doi.org/10.1515/jcim-2013-0021 Web.
12. Carrera-Quintanar, Lucrecia et al. 'Phytochemicals That Influence Gut Microbiota as Prophylactics and for the Treatment of Obesity and Inflammatory Diseases.' *Mediators of inflammation* vol. 2018 9734845. 26 Mar. 2018, doi:10.1155/2018/9734845.
13. Mahapatra, D. (Ed.), Bharti, S. (Ed.). (2019). *Medicinal Chemistry with Pharmaceutical Product Development*. New York: Apple Academic Press, https://doi.org/10.1201/9780429487842

14. Pandey, Kanti Bhooshan, and Syed Ibrahim Rizvi. 'Plant polyphenols as dietary antioxidants in human health and disease.' *Oxidative medicine and cellular longevity* vol. 2,5 (2009): 270-8. doi:10.4161/oxim.2.5.9498.
15. Midori Natsume (2018). 'Polyphenols: Inflammation'. *Current Pharmaceutical Design* 24: 191. https://doi.org/10.2174/1381612823666171109104141.
16. Hussain, T., Tan, B., Yin, Y., Blachier, F., Tossou, M. C., & Rahu, N. (2016). Oxidative Stress and Inflammation: What Polyphenols Can Do for Us?. *Oxidative medicine and cellular longevity*, *2016*, 7432797. https://doi.org/10.1155/2016/7432797.
17. Graham H. N. (1992). Green tea composition, consumption, and polyphenol chemistry. *Preventive medicine*, *21*(3), 334–350. https://doi.org/10.1016/0091-7435(92)90041-f.
18. Ahmed, S., Richard S. J. (2013). 'Chapter 2 - Green Tea: The Plants, Processing, Manufacturing and Production', *Tea in Health and Disease Prevention, Academic Press*. 19-31. https://doi.org/10.1016/B978-0-12-384937-3.00002-1.
19. Oliviero, F., Scanu, A., Zamudio-Cuevas, Y., Punzi, L., & Spinella, P. (2018). Anti-inflammatory effects of polyphenols in arthritis. *Journal of the science of food and agriculture*, *98*(5), 1653–1659. https://doi.org/10.1002/jsfa.8664.
20. Carmen Cabrera, Reyes Artacho & Rafael Giménez. (2006). Beneficial Effects of Green Tea—A Review, *Journal of the American College of Nutrition*, 25:2, 79-99, DOI: 10.1080/07315724.2006.10719518.
21. Weiss, D. J., & Anderton, C. R. (2003). Determination of catechins in matcha green tea by micellar electrokinetic chromatography. *Journal of chromatography. A*, *1011*(1-2), 173–180. https://doi.org/10.1016/s0021-9673(03)01133-6.
22. Singh, R., Akhtar, N., & Haqqi, T. M. (2010). Green tea polyphenol epigallocatechin-3-gallate: inflammation and arthritis. [corrected]. *Life sciences*, *86*(25-26), 907–918. https://doi.org/10.1016/j.lfs.2010.04.013.
23. Aggarwal, B. B., Kumar, A., & Bharti, A. C. (2003). Anticancer potential of curcumin: preclinical and clinical studies. *Anticancer research*, *23*(1A), 363–398.
24. Yang, M., Akbar, U., & Mohan, C. (2019). Curcumin in Autoimmune and Rheumatic Diseases. *Nutrients*, *11*(5), 1004. https://doi.org/10.3390/nu11051004.
25. M Khopde, S., Priyadarsini, K. I., Venkatesan, P., & Rao, M. N. (1999). Free radical scavenging ability and antioxidant efficiency of curcumin and its substituted analogue. *Biophysical chemistry*, *80*(2), 85–91. https://doi.org/10.1016/s0301-4622(99)00070-8.
26. Aggarwal, B. B., & Sung, B. (2009). Pharmacological basis for the role of curcumin in chronic diseases: an age-old spice with modern targets. *Trends*

in pharmacological sciences, *30*(2), 85–94. https://doi.org/10.1016/j.tips.2008.11.002.

27. Gupta, S. C., Patchva, S., & Aggarwal, B. B. (2013). Therapeutic roles of curcumin: lessons learned from clinical trials. *The AAPS journal*, *15*(1), 195–218. https://doi.org/10.1208/s12248-012-9432-8.
28. Aggarwal, B. B., & Harikumar, K. B. (2009). Potential therapeutic effects of curcumin, the anti-inflammatory agent, against neurodegenerative, cardiovascular, pulmonary, metabolic, autoimmune and neoplastic diseases. *The international journal of biochemistry & cell biology*, *41*(1), 40–59. https://doi.org/10.1016/j.biocel.2008.06.010.
29. Yang, M., Akbar, U., & Mohan, C. (2019). Curcumin in Autoimmune and Rheumatic Diseases. *Nutrients*, *11*(5), 1004. https://doi.org/10.3390/nu11051004.
30. Fairweather-Tait, S.J., Southon S., (2003). BIOAVAILABILITY OF NUTRIENTS, *Encyclopedia of Food Sciences and Nutrition, Elsevier: 478-484*.https://doi.org/10.1016/B0-12-227055-X/00096-1.
31. Hewlings, S. J., & Kalman, D. S. (2017). Curcumin: A Review of Its Effects on Human Health. *Foods (Basel, Switzerland)*, 6(10), 92. https://doi.org/10.3390/foods6100092.
32. Kunnumakkara, A. B., Sailo, B. L., Banik, K., Harsha, C., Prasad, S., Gupta, S. C., Bharti, A. C., & Aggarwal, B. B. (2018). Chronic diseases, inflammation, and spices: how are they linked?. *Journal of translational medicine*, *16*(1), 14. https://doi.org/10.1186/s12967-018-1381-2.
33. Umar, S., Golam Sarwar, A. H., Umar, K., Ahmad, N., Sajad, M., Ahmad, S., Katiyar, C. K., & Khan, H. A. (2013). Piperine ameliorates oxidative stress, inflammation and histological outcome in collagen induced arthritis. *Cellular immunology*, *284*(1-2), 51–59. https://doi.org/10.1016/j.cellimm.2013.07.004.
34. Semwal, R. B., Semwal, D. K., Combrinck, S., & Viljoen, A. M. (2015). Gingerols and shogaols: Important nutraceutical principles from ginger. *Phytochemistry*, *117*, 554–568. https://doi.org/10.1016/j.phytochem.2015.07.012.
35. Kumar, S., Saxena, K., Singh, U.N., Saxen, R. (2013). Anti-inflammatory action of ginger: A critical review in anemia of inflammation and its future aspects, *International Journal of Herbal Medicine, 1 (4): 16-20*. http://www.florajournal.com/archives/2013/vol1issue4/PartA/2.1.pdf.
36. Levy, A. S., Simon, O., Shelly, J., & Gardener, M. (2006). 6-Shogaol reduced chronic inflammatory response in the knees of rats treated with complete Freund's adjuvant. *BMC Pharmacology*, 6, 12. https://doi.org/10.1186/1471-2210-6-12.

37. Sharma, J. N., Srivastava, K. C., & Gan, E. K. (1994). Suppressive effects of eugenol and ginger oil on arthritic rats. *Pharmacology*, *49*(5), 314–318. https://doi.org/10.1159/000139248.
38. Funk, J. L., Frye, J. B., Oyarzo, J. N., & Timmermann, B. N. (2009). Comparative effects of two gingerol-containing *Zingiber officinale* extracts on experimental rheumatoid arthritis. *Journal of natural products*, *72*(3), 403–407. https://doi.org/10.1021/np8006183.
39. Pragasam, S.J., Kumar, S., Bhoumik, M., Sabina, E. P., Rasool, M. (2011). '6-Gingerol, an active ingredient of ginger suppresses monosodium ureate crystal-induced inflammation: an in vivo and in vitro evaluation,' *Annals of Biological Research, 2(3),* 200–208.
40. Srivastava, K. C., & Mustafa, T. (1992). Ginger (*Zingiber officinale*) in rheumatism and musculoskeletal disorders. *Medical hypotheses*, *39*(4), 342–348. https://doi.org/10.1016/0306-9877(92)90059-l.
41. Srivastava, K. C., & Mustafa, T. (1992). Ginger (*Zingiber officinale*) in rheumatism and musculoskeletal disorders. *Medical hypotheses*, *39*(4), 342–348. https://doi.org/10.1016/0306-9877(92)90059-l.
42. Altman, R. D., & Marcussen, K. C. (2001). Effects of a ginger extract on knee pain in patients with osteoarthritis. *Arthritis and rheumatism*, *44*(11), 2531–2538. https://doi.org/10.1002/1529-0131(200111)44:11<2531::aid-art433>3.0.co;2-j.
43. Haghighi M, Khalvat A, Toliat T, Jallaei S. (2005). Comparing the Effects of Ginger (*Zingiber officinale*) Extract and Ibuprofen on Patients with Osteoarthritis. *Arch Iran Med*. 8(4):267–71.
44. Aryaeian, N., Mahmoudi, M., Shahram, F., Poursani, S., Jamshidi, F., & Tavakoli, H. (2019). The effect of ginger supplementation on IL2, TNFα, and IL1β cytokines gene expression levels in patients with active rheumatoid arthritis: A randomized controlled trial. *Medical journal of the Islamic Republic of Iran*, *33*, 154. https://doi.org/10.34171/mjiri.33.154.
45. Yoshikawa, M., Hatakeyama, S., Chatani, N., Nishino, Y., & Yamahara, J. (1993). *Yakugaku zasshi : Journal of the Pharmaceutical Society of Japan*, *113*(4), 307–315. https://doi.org/10.1248/yakushi1947.113.4_307.
46. Aryaeian, N., Mahmoudi, M., Shahram, F., Poursani, S., Jamshidi, F., & Tavakoli, H. (2019). The effect of ginger supplementation on IL2, TNFα, and IL1β cytokines gene expression levels in patients with active rheumatoid arthritis: A randomized controlled trial. *Medical journal of the Islamic Republic of Iran*, *33*, 154. https://doi.org/10.34171/mjiri.33.154.
47. Aryaeian, N., Shahram, F., Mahmoudi, M., Tavakoli, H., Yousefi, B., Arablou, T., & Jafari Karegar, S. (2019). The effect of ginger supplementation on some immunity and inflammation intermediate genes expression

in patients with active Rheumatoid Arthritis. *Gene*, *698*, 179–185. https://doi.org/10.1016/j.gene.2019.01.048.

48. Ramadan, G., Al-Kahtani, M. A., & El-Sayed, W. M. (2011). Anti-inflammatory and anti-oxidant properties of *Curcuma longa* (turmeric) versus *Zingiber officinale* (ginger) rhizomes in rat adjuvant-induced arthritis. *Inflammation*, *34*(4), 291–301. https://doi.org/10.1007/s10753-010-9278-0.
49. Prasad S, Aggarwal BB. (2014). Chronic Diseases Caused by Chronic Inflammation Require Chronic Treatment: Anti-inflammatory Role of Dietary Spices. *J Clin Cell Immunol 5: 238*. doi:10.4172/2155-9899.1000238.
50. Rehman R., Akram M, Akhtar N., et al. (2001). *Zingiber officinale* roscoe (pharmacological activity). *J Med Plant Res. 5(3):344-348*.
51. Zakeri Z., Izadi S., Bari Z., Soltani F., Narouie B., Rad M.G. (2011). Evaluating the effects of ginger extract on knee pain, stiffness and difficulty in patients with knee osteoarthritis. *Journal of Medicinal Plants Research. 5(15)*:3375-3379. https://academicjournals.org/article/article1380629850_Zakeri%20et%20al.pdf
52. Feng T., Su J., Ding Z.H., et al. (2001). Chemical constituents and their bioactivities of 'Tongling white ginger' (Zingiber officinale). *J Agric Food Chem. 9(21)*:11690-11695. doi: 10.1021/jf202544w.
53. Santangelo, C., Vari, R., Scazzocchio, B., De Sanctis, P., Giovannini, C., D'Archivio, M., & Masella, R. (2018). Anti-inflammatory Activity of Extra Virgin Olive Oil Polyphenols: Which Role in the Prevention and Treatment of Immune-Mediated Inflammatory Diseases?. *Endocrine, metabolic & immune disorders drug targets*, *18*(1), 36–50. https://doi.org/10.2174/1871530317666171114114321.
54. Vilaplana-Pérez, C., Auñón, D., García-Flores, L. A., & Gil-Izquierdo, A. (2014). Hydroxytyrosol and potential uses in cardiovascular diseases, cancer, and AIDS. *Frontiers in nutrition*, *1*, 18. https://doi.org/10.3389/fnut.2014.00018
55. EFSA Panel on Dietetic Products, Nutrition and Allergies (NDA). (2011). Scientific Opinion on the substantiation of health claims related to polyphenols in olive and protection of LDL particles from oxidative damage, *EFSA Journal,* 9(4):2033. doi:10.2903/j.efsa.2011.2033. Available online: www.efsa.europa.eu/efsajournal.
56. Santangelo, C., Vari, R., Scazzocchio, B., De Sanctis, P., Giovannini, C., D'Archivio, M., & Masella, R. (2018). Anti-inflammatory Activity of Extra Virgin Olive Oil Polyphenols: Which Role in the Prevention and Treatment of Immune-Mediated Inflammatory Diseases?. *Endocrine, metabolic & immune disorders drug targets*, *18*(1), 36–50. https://doi.org/10.2174/1871530317666171114114321.

57. Aparicio-Soto, M., Sánchez-Hidalgo, M., Rosillo, M. Á., Castejón, M. L., & Alarcón-de-la-Lastra, C. (2016). Extra virgin olive oil: a key functional food for prevention of immune-inflammatory diseases. *Food & function*, 7(11), 4492–4505. https://doi.org/10.1039/c6fo01094f.
58. Santangelo, C., Vari, R., Scazzocchio, B., De Sanctis, P., Giovannini, C., D'Archivio, M., & Masella, R. (2018). Anti-inflammatory Activity of Extra Virgin Olive Oil Polyphenols: Which Role in the Prevention and Treatment of Immune-Mediated Inflammatory Diseases?. *Endocrine, metabolic & immune disorders drug targets*, *18*(1), 36–50. https://doi.org/10.2174/1871530317666171114114321.
59. Aparicio-Soto, M., Sánchez-Hidalgo, M., Rosillo, M. Á., Castejón, M. L., & Alarcón-de-la-Lastra, C. (2016). Extra virgin olive oil: a key functional food for prevention of immune-inflammatory diseases. *Food & function*, 7(11), 4492–4505. https://doi.org/10.1039/c6fo01094f.
60. Ángeles, M.R., Sánchez-Hidalgo, M., Castejón, M.L, Montoya, T., González-Benjumea, A., Fernández-Bolaños, J,G., Alarcón-de-la-Lastra, C. (2017). Extra-virgin olive oil phenols hydroxytyrosol and hydroxytyrosol acetate, down-regulate the production of mediators involved in joint erosion in human synovial cells, *Journal of Functional Foods*, 36, 27-33, https://doi.org/10.1016/j.jff.2017.06.041.
61. Aparicio-Soto, M., Sánchez-Hidalgo, M., Rosillo, M. Á., Castejón, M. L., & Alarcón-de-la-Lastra, C. (2016). Extra virgin olive oil: a key functional food for prevention of immune-inflammatory diseases. *Food & function*, 7(11), 4492–4505. https://doi.org/10.1039/c6fo01094f.
62. Vinitha, M., Ballal, M., 2008. In vitro Anticandidal Activity of *Cinnamomum verum*. *Journal of Medical Sciences*, 8: 425-428, doi: 10.3923/jms.2008.425.428.
63. Rathi, B., Bodhankar, S., Mohan, V., & Thakurdesai, P. (2013). Ameliorative Effects of a Polyphenolic Fraction of *Cinnamomum zeylanicum* L. Bark in Animal Models of Inflammation and Arthritis. *Scientia pharmaceutica*, *81*(2), 567–589. https://doi.org/10.3797/scipharm.1301-16.
64. Gruenwald, J., Freder, J., & Armbruester, N. (2010). Cinnamon and health. *Critical reviews in food science and nutrition*, *50*(9), 822–834. https://doi.org/10.1080/10408390902773052.
65. Rathi, B., Bodhankar, S., Mohan, V., & Thakurdesai, P. (2013). Ameliorative Effects of a Polyphenolic Fraction of *Cinnamomum zeylanicum* L. Bark in Animal Models of Inflammation and Arthritis. *Scientia pharmaceutica*, *81*(2), 567–589. https://doi.org/10.3797/scipharm.1301-16 .
66. Kunnumakkara, A. B., Sailo, B. L., Banik, K., Harsha, C., Prasad, S., Gupta, S. C., Bharti, A. C., & Aggarwal, B. B. (2018). Chronic diseases,

inflammation, and spices: how are they linked?. *Journal of translational medicine*, *16*(1), 14. https://doi.org/10.1186/s12967-018-1381-2.

67. Shishehbor, F., Rezaeyan Safar, M., Rajaei, E., & Haghighizadeh, M. H. (2018). Cinnamon Consumption Improves Clinical Symptoms and Inflammatory Markers in Women With Rheumatoid Arthritis. *Journal of the American College of Nutrition*, 1–6. Advance online publication. https://doi.org/10.1080/07315724.2018.1460733.
68. Vázquez-Fresno, R., Rosana, A., Sajed, T., Onookome-Okome, T., Wishart, N. A., & Wishart, D. S. (2019). Herbs and Spices- Biomarkers of Intake Based on Human Intervention Studies - A Systematic Review. *Genes & nutrition*, *14*, 18. https://doi.org/10.1186/s12263-019-0636-8.
69. Ghorbani, A., & Esmaeilizadeh, M. (2017). Pharmacological properties of *Salvia officinalis* and its components. *Journal of traditional and complementary medicine*, 7(4), 433–440. https://doi.org/10.1016/j.jtcme.2016.12.014.
70. López-Jiménez, A., García-Caballero, M., Medina, M. Á., & Quesada, A. R. (2013). Anti-angiogenic properties of carnosol and carnosic acid, two major dietary compounds from rosemary. *European journal of nutrition*, *52*(1), 85–95. https://doi.org/10.1007/s00394-011-0289-x.
71. Sanchez, C., Horcajada, M. N., Membrez Scalfo, F., Ameye, L., Offord, E., & Henrotin, Y. (2015). Carnosol Inhibits Pro-Inflammatory and Catabolic Mediators of Cartilage Breakdown in Human Osteoarthritic Chondrocytes and Mediates Cross-Talk between Subchondral Bone Osteoblasts and Chondrocytes. *PloS one*, *10*(8), e0136118. https://doi.org/10.1371/journal.pone.0136118.
72. Wang, J., Yang, G., Hua, Y., Sun, T., Gao, C., Xia, Q., Li, B. (2016). Carnosol ameliorates monosodium iodoacetate-induced osteoarthritis by targeting NF-κB and Nrf-2 in primary rat chondrocytes, *Journal of Applied Biomedicine,14(4):* 307-314, https://doi.org/10.1016/j.jab.2016.05.001.
73. Schwager, J., Richard, N., Fowler, A., Seifert, N., & Raederstorff, D. (2016). Carnosol and Related Substances Modulate Chemokine and Cytokine Production in Macrophages and Chondrocytes. *Molecules (Basel, Switzerland)*, *21*(4), 465. https://doi.org/10.3390/molecules21040465.
74. Xia, G., Wang, X., Sun, H., Qin, Y., & Fu, M. (2017). Carnosic acid (CA) attenuates collagen-induced arthritis in db/db mice via inflammation suppression by regulating ROS-dependent p38 pathway. *Free radical biology & medicine*, *108*, 418–432. https://doi.org/10.1016/j.freeradbiomed.2017.03.023.
75. Poeckel, D., Greiner, C., Verhoff, M., Rau, O., Tausch, L., Hörnig, C., Steinhilber, D., Schubert-Zsilavecz, M., & Werz, O. (2008). Carnosic

acid and carnosol potently inhibit human 5-lipoxygenase and suppress pro-inflammatory responses of stimulated human polymorphonuclear leukocytes. *Biochemical pharmacology*, 76(1), 91–97. https://doi.org/10.1016/j.bcp.2008.04.013.

76. Lo, A. H., Liang, Y. C., Lin-Shiau, S. Y., Ho, C. T., & Lin, J. K. (2002). Carnosol, an antioxidant in rosemary, suppresses inducible nitric oxide synthase through down-regulating nuclear factor-kappaB in mouse macrophages. *Carcinogenesis*, *23*(6), 983–991. https://doi.org/10.1093/carcin/23.6.983.
77. Soleas, G. J., Diamandis, E. P., & Goldberg, D. M. (1997). Wine as a biological fluid: history, production, and role in disease prevention. *Journal of clinical laboratory analysis*, *11*(5), 287–313. https://doi.org/10.1002/(SICI)1098-2825(1997)11:5<287::AID-JCLA6>3.0.CO;2-4.
78. Kuršvietienė, L., Stanevičienė, I., Mongirdienė, A., & Bernatonienė, J. (2016). Multiplicity of effects and health benefits of resveratrol. *Medicina (Kaunas, Lithuania)*, 52(3), 148–155. https://doi.org/10.1016/j.medici.2016.03.003.
79. Bertelli, A. A., Ferrara, F., Diana, G., Fulgenzi, A., Corsi, M., Ponti, W., Ferrero, M. E., & Bertelli, A. (1999). Resveratrol, a natural stilbene in grapes and wine, enhances intraphagocytosis in human promonocytes: a co-factor in anti-inflammatory and anticancer chemopreventive activity. *International journal of tissue reactions*, *21*(4), 93–104.
80. Nguyen, C., Savouret, J. F., Widerak, M., Corvol, M. T., & Rannou, F. (2017). Resveratrol, Potential Therapeutic Interest in Joint Disorders: A Critical Narrative Review. *Nutrients*, 9(1), 45. https://doi.org/10.3390/nu9010045.
81. Riveiro-Naveira, R.R. & Loureiro, Jesús & Valcarcel-Ares, M. Noa & López-Peláez, E. & Cortes, Alberto & Vaamonde-García, Carlos & Hermida-Carballo, L. & Blanco, Francisco & López-Armada, María. (2014). Anti-inflammatory effect of resveratrol as a dietary supplement in an antigen-induced arthritis rat model. *Osteoarthritis and Cartilage*. 22. S290. 10.1016/j.joca.2014.02.539. https://www.oarsijournal.com/article/S1063-4584(14)00579-2/pdf.
82. Wei, Y., Jia, J., Jin, X., Tong, W., & Tian, H. (2018). Resveratrol ameliorates inflammatory damage and protects against osteoarthritis in a rat model of osteoarthritis. *Molecular medicine reports*, *17*(1), 1493–1498. https://doi.org/10.3892/mmr.2017.8036.
83. Marouf, B. H., Hussain, S. A., Ali, Z. S., & Ahmmad, R. S. (2018). Resveratrol Supplementation Reduces Pain and Inflammation in Knee Osteoarthritis Patients Treated with Meloxicam: A Randomized Placebo-Controlled Study. *Journal of medicinal food*, 10.1089/jmf.2017.4176.

84. Elmali, N., Baysal, O., Harma, A., Esenkaya, I., & Mizrak, B. (2007). Effects of resveratrol in inflammatory arthritis. *Inflammation*, *30*(1-2), 1–6. https://doi.org/10.1007/s10753-006-9012-0.
85. Khojah, H. M., Ahmed, S., Abdel-Rahman, M. S., & Elhakeim, E. H. (2018). Resveratrol as an effective adjuvant therapy in the management of rheumatoid arthritis: a clinical study. *Clinical rheumatology*, *37*(8), 2035–2042. https://doi.org/10.1007/s10067-018-4080-8.
86. Cruz Rosas, E., Barbosa Correa, L., das Graças Henriques, M. (2019). Chapter 28 - Anti-inflammatory Properties of *Schinus terebinthifolius* and Its Use in Arthritic Conditions, *Bioactive Food as Dietary Interventions for Arthritis and Related Inflammatory Diseases (Second Edition)*, 489-505, https://doi.org/10.1016/B978-0-12-813820-5.00028-3.
87. Pan, D., Li, N., Liu, Y., Xu, Q., Liu, Q., You, Y., Wei, Z., Jiang, Y., Liu, M., Guo, T., Cai, X., Liu, X., Wang, Q., Liu, M., Lei, X., Zhang, M., Zhao, X., & Lin, C. (2018). Kaempferol inhibits the migration and invasion of rheumatoid arthritis fibroblast-like synoviocytes by blocking activation of the MAPK pathway. *International immunopharmacology*, *55*, 174–182. https://doi.org/10.1016/j.intimp.2017.12.011.
88. Lin, F., Luo, X., Tsun, A., Li, Z., Li, D., & Li, B. (2015). Kaempferol enhances the suppressive function of Treg cells by inhibiting FOXP3 phosphorylation. *International immunopharmacology*, *28*(2), 859–865. https://doi.org/10.1016/j.intimp.2015.03.044.
89. Jiang, R., Hao, P., Yu, G., Liu, C., Yu, C., Huang, Y., & Wang, Y. (2019). Kaempferol protects chondrogenic ATDC5 cells against inflammatory injury triggered by lipopolysaccharide through down-regulating miR-146a. *International immunopharmacology*, *69*, 373–381. https://doi.org/10.1016/j.intimp.2019.02.014.
90. Zhuang, Z., Ye, G., & Huang, B. (2017). Kaempferol Alleviates the Interleukin-1β-Induced Inflammation in Rat Osteoarthritis Chondrocytes via Suppression of NF-κB. *Medical science monitor: international medical journal of experimental and clinical research*, *23*, 3925–3931. https://doi.org/10.12659/msm.902491.
91. Li, J., Gang, D., Yu, X., Hu, Y., Yue, Y., Cheng, W., Pan, X., & Zhang, P. (2013). Genistein: the potential for efficacy in rheumatoid arthritis. *Clinical rheumatology*, *32*(5), 535–540. https://doi.org/10.1007/s10067-012-2148-4.
92. Li, J., Li, J., Yue, Y., Hu, Y., Cheng, W., Liu, R., Pan, X., & Zhang, P. (2014). Genistein suppresses tumor necrosis factor α-induced inflammation via modulating reactive oxygen species/Akt/nuclear factor κB and adenosine monophosphate-activated protein kinase signal pathways in human

synoviocyte MH7A cells. *Drug design, development and therapy*, *8*, 315–323. https://doi.org/10.2147/DDDT.S52354.

93. Xu, J. X., Zhang, Y., Zhang, X. Z., & Ma, Y. Y. (2011). *Zhong xi yi jie he xue bao = Journal of Chinese integrative medicine*, *9*(2), 186–193. https://doi.org/10.3736/jcim20110212.
94. Valsecchi, A. E., Franchi, S., Panerai, A. E., Sacerdote, P., Trovato, A. E., & Colleoni, M. (2008). Genistein, a natural phytoestrogen from soy, relieves neuropathic pain following chronic constriction sciatic nerve injury in mice: anti-inflammatory and antioxidant activity. *Journal of neurochemistry*, *107*(1), 230–240. https://doi.org/10.1111/j.1471-4159.2008.05614.x.
95. Liu, F. C., Wang, C. C., Lu, J. W., Lee, C. H., Chen, S. C., Ho, Y. J., & Peng, Y. J. (2019). Chondroprotective Effects of Genistein against Osteoarthritis Induced Joint Inflammation. *Nutrients*, *11*(5), 1180. https://doi.org/10.3390/nu11051180.
96. Bischoff S. C. (2008). Quercetin: potentials in the prevention and therapy of disease. *Current opinion in clinical nutrition and metabolic care*, *11*(6), 733–740. https://doi.org/10.1097/MCO.0b013e32831394b8.
97. Mitchell, A. E., Hong, Y. J., Koh, E., Barrett, D. M., Bryant, D. E., Denison, R. F., & Kaffka, S. (2007). Ten-year comparison of the influence of organic and conventional crop management practices on the content of flavonoids in tomatoes. *Journal of agricultural and food chemistry*, *55*(15), 6154–6159. https://doi.org/10.1021/jf070344+.
98. Gardi, C., Bauerova, K., Stringa, B., Kuncirova, V., Slovak, L., Ponist, S., Drafi, F., Bezakova, L., Tedesco, I., Acquaviva, A., Bilotto, S., & Russo, G. L. (2015). Quercetin reduced inflammation and increased antioxidant defense in rat adjuvant arthritis. *Archives of biochemistry and biophysics*, *583*, 150–157. https://doi.org/10.1016/j.abb.2015.08.008.
99. García-Mediavilla, V., Crespo, I., Collado, P. S., Esteller, A., Sánchez-Campos, S., Tuñón, M. J., & González-Gallego, J. (2007). The anti-inflammatory flavones quercetin and kaempferol cause inhibition of inducible nitric oxide synthase, cyclooxygenase-2 and reactive C-protein, and down-regulation of the nuclear factor kappaB pathway in Chang Liver cells. *European journal of pharmacology*, *557*(2-3), 221–229. https://doi.org/10.1016/j.ejphar.2006.11.014.
100. Anand David, A. V., Arulmoli, R., & Parasuraman, S. (2016). Overviews of Biological Importance of Quercetin: A Bioactive Flavonoid. *Pharmacognosy reviews*, *10*(20), 84–89. https://doi.org/10.4103/0973-7847.194044.
101. Guardia, T., Rotelli, A. E., Juarez, A. O., & Pelzer, L. E. (2001). Anti-inflammatory properties of plant flavonoids. Effects of rutin, quercetin and hesperidin on adjuvant arthritis in rat. *Farmaco (Societa chimica italiana : 1989)*, *56*(9), 683–687. https://doi.org/10.1016/s0014-827x(01)01111-9.

102. Mamani-Matsuda, M., Kauss, T., Al-Kharrat, A., Rambert, J., Fawaz, F., Thiolat, D., Moynet, D., Coves, S., Malvy, D., & Mossalayi, M. D. (2006). Therapeutic and preventive properties of quercetin in experimental arthritis correlate with decreased macrophage inflammatory mediators. *Biochemical pharmacology*, *72*(10), 1304–1310. https://doi.org/10.1016/j.bcp.2006.08.001.
103. Salgado, R., P., Di Giorgio, L., Musso, S.,Y., Mauri, A.,N., (2019). Chapter 9 - Bioactive Packaging: Combining Nanotechnologies With Packaging for Improved Food Functionality, In Micro and Nano Technologies, *Nanomaterials for Food Applications,* 233-270, https://doi.org/10.1016/B978-0-12-814130-4.00009-9.
104. Liu, W., Zhang, L., Xu, H. J., Li, Y., Hu, C. M., Yang, J. Y., & Sun, M. Y. (2018). The Anti-Inflammatory Effects of Vitamin D in Tumorigenesis. *International journal of molecular sciences*, *19*(9), 2736. https://doi.org/10.3390/ijms19092736.
105. Salgado, R., P., Di Giorgio, L., Musso, S.,Y., Mauri, A.,N., (2019). Chapter 9 - Bioactive Packaging: Combining Nanotechnologies With Packaging for Improved Food Functionality, In Micro and Nano Technologies, *Nanomaterials for Food Applications,* 233-270, https://doi.org/10.1016/B978-0-12-814130-4.00009-9.
106. Palacios, C., & Gonzalez, L. (2014). Is vitamin D deficiency a major global public health problem?. *The Journal of steroid biochemistry and molecular biology*, *144 Pt A*, 138–145. https://doi.org/10.1016/j.jsbmb.2013.11.003.
107. Kostoglou-Athanassiou, I., Athanassiou, P., Lyraki, A., Raftakis, I., & Antoniadis, C. (2012). Vitamin D and rheumatoid arthritis. *Therapeutic advances in endocrinology and metabolism*, *3*(6), 181–187. https://doi.org/10.1177/2042018812471070.
108. McAlindon, T. E., Felson, D. T., Zhang, Y., Hannan, M. T., Aliabadi, P., Weissman, B., Rush, D., Wilson, P. W., & Jacques, P. (1996). Relation of dietary intake and serum levels of vitamin D to progression of osteoarthritis of the knee among participants in the Framingham Study. *Annals of internal medicine*, *125*(5), 353–359. https://doi.org/10.7326/0003-4819-125-5-199609010-00001.
109. Bergink, A. P., Uitterlinden, A. G., Van Leeuwen, J. P., Buurman, C. J., Hofman, A., Verhaar, J. A., & Pols, H. A. (2009). Vitamin D status, bone mineral density, and the development of radiographic osteoarthritis of the knee: The Rotterdam Study. *Journal of clinical rheumatology : practical reports on rheumatic & musculoskeletal diseases*, *15*(5), 230–237. https://doi.org/10.1097/RHU.0b013e3181b08f20.

110. Heidari, B., Heidari, P., & Hajian-Tilaki, K. (2011). Association between serum vitamin D deficiency and knee osteoarthritis. *International orthopaedics*, *35*(11), 1627–1631. https://doi.org/10.1007/s00264-010-1186-2.
111. Manoy, P., Yuktanandana, P., Tanavalee, A., Anomasiri, W., Ngarmukos, S., Tanpowpong, T., & Honsawek, S. (2017). Vitamin D Supplementation Improves Quality of Life and Physical Performance in Osteoarthritis Patients. *Nutrients*, *9*(8), 799. https://doi.org/10.3390/nu9080799.
112. Ross, A., C., Taylor, C., L., Yaktine A., L., (2011). 3, Overview of Vitamin D. *Institute of Medicine (US) Committee to Review Dietary Reference Intakes for Vitamin D and Calcium. Dietary Reference Intakes for Calcium and Vitamin D.* https://www.ncbi.nlm.nih.gov/books/NBK56061/
113. Young, A., Narbutt, J., Harrison, G., Lawrence, K., Bell, M., O'Connor, C., Olsen, P., Grys, K., Baczynska, K., Rogowski-Tylman, M., Wulf, H., Lesiak, A. and Philipsen, P. (2019), Optimal sunscreen use, during a sun holiday with a very high ultraviolet index, allows vitamin D synthesis without sunburn. *Br J Dermatol, 181:* 1052-1062. doi:10.1111/bjd.17888.
114. Mohania, D., Chandel, S., Kumar, P., Verma, V., Digvijay, K., Tripathi, D., Choudhury, K., Mitten, S. K., & Shah, D. (2017). Ultraviolet Radiations: Skin Defense-Damage Mechanism. *Advances in experimental medicine and biology*, *996*, 71–87. https://doi.org/10.1007/978-3-319-56017-5_7.
115. Australian Government, (2012), Focus on Kakadu Plum, *The Rural Industries Research & Development Corporation (RIRDC)*, https://www.agrifutures.com.au/wp-content/uploads/publications/14-115.pdf.
116. Arablou T, Aryaeian N, Djalali M, Shahram F, Rasouli L., (2019). Association between dietary intake of some antioxidant micronutrients with some inflammatory and antioxidant markers in active Rheumatoid Arthritis patients. *Int J Vitam Nutr Res*. 89(5-6):238-245. doi:10.1024/0300-9831/a000255.
117. Lindsey, R. C., Cheng, S., & Mohan, S. (2019). Vitamin C effects on 5-hydroxymethylcytosine and gene expression in osteoblasts and chondrocytes: Potential involvement of PHD2. *PloS one*, *14*(8), e0220653.
118. Chiu, P. R., Hu, Y. C., Huang, T. C., Hsieh, B. S., Yeh, J. P., Cheng, H. L., Huang, L. W., & Chang, K. L. (2016). Vitamin C Protects Chondrocytes against Monosodium Iodoacetate-Induced Osteoarthritis by Multiple Pathways. *International journal of molecular sciences*, *18*(1), 38. https://doi.org/10.3390/ijms18010038.
119. Joseph, G. B., McCulloch, C. E., Nevitt, M. C., Neumann, J., Lynch, J. A., Lane, N. E., & Link, T. M. (2020). Associations Between Vitamins C and D Intake and Cartilage Composition and Knee Joint Morphology Over 4 Years: Data From the Osteoarthritis Initiative. *Arthritis care & research*, *72*(9), 1239–1247. https://doi.org/10.1002/acr.24021.

120. Juraschek, S. P., Miller, E. R., 3rd, & Gelber, A. C. (2011). Effect of oral vitamin C supplementation on serum uric acid: a meta-analysis of randomized controlled trials. *Arthritis care & research*, *63*(9), 1295–1306. https://doi.org/10.1002/acr.20519.
121. Carr, A. C., & McCall, C. (2017). The role of vitamin C in the treatment of pain: new insights. *Journal of translational medicine*, *15*(1), 77. https://doi.org/10.1186/s12967-017-1179-7.
122. Pattison, D. J., Silman, A. J., Goodson, N. J., Lunt, M., Bunn, D., Luben, R., Welch, A., Bingham, S., Khaw, K. T., Day, N., & Symmons, D. P. (2004). Vitamin C and the risk of developing inflammatory polyarthritis: prospective nested case-control study. *Annals of the rheumatic diseases*, *63*(7), 843–847. https://doi.org/10.1136/ard.2003.016097.
123. Salgado, R., P., Di Giorgio, L., Musso, S.,Y., Mauri, A.,N., (2019). Chapter 9 - Bioactive Packaging: Combining Nanotechnologies With Packaging for Improved Food Functionality, In Micro and Nano Technologies, *Nanomaterials for Food Applications,* 233-270, https://doi.org/10.1016/B978-0-12-814130-4.00009-9.
124. O'Dell, J. R., Lemley-Gillespie, S., Palmer, W. R., Weaver, A. L., Moore, G. F., & Klassen, L. W. (1991). Serum selenium concentrations in rheumatoid arthritis. *Annals of the rheumatic diseases*, *50*(6), 376–378. https://doi.org/10.1136/ard.50.6.376.
125. Yu, N., Han, F., Lin, X., Tang, C., Ye, J., & Cai, X. (2016). The Association Between Serum Selenium Levels with Rheumatoid Arthritis. *Biological trace element research*, *172*(1), 46–52. https://doi.org/10.1007/s12011-015-0558-2.
126. University of North Carolina at Chapel Hill. (2005). Study Links Low Selenium Levels With Higher Risk Of Osteoarthritis. *ScienceDaily*. Retrieved August 14, 2020 from www.sciencedaily.com/releases/2005/11/051114112959.htm.
127. Hasani, M., Djalalinia, S., Khazdooz, M., Asayesh, H., Zarei, M., Gorabi, A. M., Ansari, H., Qorbani, M., & Heshmat, R. (2019). Effect of selenium supplementation on antioxidant markers: a systematic review and meta-analysis of randomized controlled trials. *Hormones (Athens, Greece)*, *18*(4), 451–462. https://doi.org/10.1007/s42000-019-00143-3.
128. Deyab, G., Hokstad, I., Aaseth, J., Småstuen, M. C., Whist, J. E., Agewall, S., Lyberg, T., Tveiten, D., Hjeltnes, G., Zibara, K., & Hollan, I. (2018). Effect of anti-rheumatic treatment on selenium levels in inflammatory arthritis. *Journal of trace elements in medicine and biology : organ of the Society for Minerals and Trace Elements (GMS)*, *49*, 91–97. https://doi.org/10.1016/j.jtemb.2018.05.001.
129. Kohlmeier, M. (2003). Selenium, *Food Science and Technology, Nutrient Metabolism*, 722-728, https://doi.org/10.1016/B978-012417762-8.50103-4.

130. U.S. Department of Health & Human Services. (2020, March 11). Selenium Fact Sheet for Health Professionals, *National Institutes of Health: Office of Dietary Supplements*. https://ods.od.nih.gov/factsheets/Selenium-HealthProfessional/. Accessed 15.08.2020.
131. Lim, K. H., Riddell, L. J., Nowson, C. A., Booth, A. O., & Szymlek-Gay, E. A. (2013). Iron and zinc nutrition in the economically-developed world: a review. *Nutrients*, *5*(8), 3184–3211. https://doi.org/10.3390/nu5083184.
132. Sanna, A., Firinu, D., Zavattari, P., & Valera, P. (2018). Zinc Status and Autoimmunity: A Systematic Review and Meta-Analysis. *Nutrients*, *10*(1), 68. https://doi.org/10.3390/nu10010068.
133. Jarosz, M., Olbert, M., Wyszogrodzka, G., Młyniec, K., & Librowski, T. (2017). Antioxidant and anti-inflammatory effects of zinc. Zinc-dependent NF-κB signaling. *Inflammopharmacology*, *25*(1), 11–24. https://doi.org/10.1007/s10787-017-0309-4.
134. Rajaee, E., Mowla, K., Ghorbani, A. (2018). The relationship between serum zinc levels and rheumatoid arthritis activity. *Front. Biol.* 13, 51–55. https://doi.org/10.1007/s11515-017-1474-y.
135. Sanna, A., Firinu, D., Zavattari, P., & Valera, P. (2018). Zinc Status and Autoimmunity: A Systematic Review and Meta-Analysis. *Nutrients*, *10*(1), 68. https://doi.org/10.3390/nu10010068.
136. Singh, M., & Das, R. R. (2011). Zinc for the common cold. *The Cochrane database of systematic reviews*, (2), CD001364. https://doi.org/10.1002/14651858.CD001364.pub3.
137. Hemilä, H., Fitzgerald, J. T., Petrus, E. J., & Prasad, A. (2017). Zinc Acetate Lozenges May Improve the Recovery Rate of Common Cold Patients: An Individual Patient Data Meta-Analysis. *Open forum infectious diseases*, *4*(2), ofx059. https://doi.org/10.1093/ofid/ofx059.
138. Volpe S., L., (2012). Magnesium. *Present Knowledge in Nutrition.10:*459-74.
139. Gröber, U., Schmidt, J., & Kisters, K. (2015). Magnesium in Prevention and Therapy. *Nutrients*, 7(9), 8199–8226. https://doi.org/10.3390/nu7095388.
140. Tam, M., Gómez, S., González-Gross, M., & Marcos, A. (2003). Possible roles of magnesium on the immune system. *European journal of clinical nutrition*, *57*(10), 1193–1197. https://doi.org/10.1038/sj.ejcn.1601689.
141. Jahnen-Dechent, W., & Ketteler, M. (2012). Magnesium basics. *Clinical kidney journal*, *5*(Suppl 1), i3–i14. https://doi.org/10.1093/ndtplus/sfr163.
142. Nielsen, F. H., Johnson, L. K., & Zeng, H. (2010). Magnesium supplementation improves indicators of low magnesium status and inflammatory stress in adults older than 51 years with poor quality sleep. *Magnesium research*, *23*(4), 158–168. https://doi.org/10.1684/mrh.2010.0220.

143. Chandrasekaran, N. C., Weir, C., Alfraji, S., Grice, J., Roberts, M. S., & Barnard, R. T. (2014). Effects of magnesium deficiency--more than skin deep. *Experimental biology and medicine (Maywood, N.J.)*, *239*(10), 1280–1291. https://doi.org/10.1177/1535370214537745.
144. Abbasi, B., Kimiagar, M., Sadeghniiat, K., Shirazi, M. M., Hedayati, M., & Rashidkhani, B. (2012). The effect of magnesium supplementation on primary insomnia in elderly: A double-blind placebo-controlled clinical trial. *Journal of research in medical sciences : the official journal of Isfahan University of Medical Sciences*, *17*(12), 1161–1169.
145. Peuhkuri, K., Sihvola, N., & Korpela, R. (2012). Dietary factors and fluctuating levels of melatonin. *Food & nutrition research*, *56*, 10.3402/fnr.v56i0.17252. https://doi.org/10.3402/fnr.v56i0.17252.
146. Meng, X., Li, Y., Li, S., Zhou, Y., Gan, R. Y., Xu, D. P., & Li, H. B. (2017). Dietary Sources and Bioactivities of Melatonin. *Nutrients*, *9*(4), 367. https://doi.org/10.3390/nu9040367.
147. Wienecke, E., & Nolden, C. (2016). Langzeit-HRV-Analyse zeigt Stressreduktion durch Magnesiumzufuhr [Long-term HRV analysis shows stress reduction by magnesium intake]. *MMW Fortschritte der Medizin*, *158*(Suppl 6), 12–16. https://doi.org/10.1007/s15006-016-9054-7.
148. Sukenik, S., Neumann, L., Buskila, D., Kleiner-Baumgarten, A., Zimlichman, S., & Horowitz, J. (1990). Dead Sea bath salts for the treatment of rheumatoid arthritis. *Clinical and experimental rheumatology*, *8*(4), 353–357.
149. Shmagel, A., Onizuka, N., Langsetmo, L., Vo, T., Foley, R., Ensrud, K., & Valen, P. (2018). Low magnesium intake is associated with increased knee pain in subjects with radiographic knee osteoarthritis: data from the Osteoarthritis Initiative. *Osteoarthritis and cartilage*, *26*(5), 651–658. https://doi.org/10.1016/j.joca.2018.02.002.
150. Amudha G. (2014). *Assess the effectiveness of hot water compress with Epsom salt among elderly women with knee joint pain residing at selected urban area choolai in chennai* (College of Nursing Madras Medical College, Chennai – 03.) [Dissertation, The Tamilnadu Dr.M.G.R. Medical University, Chennai – 600 032.]. M. Sc (Nursing) Degree Examination Branch –Iv Community Health Nursing. https://core.ac.uk/download/pdf/235669163.pdf.
151. Sabitha, M. (2018). Evaluate the effectiveness of hot foot bath with Epsom salt on joint pain, stiffness, and physical function among patients with osteoarthritis in selected hospitals at Ottanchathiram.
152. Yang, C., Daoping, Z., Xiaoping, X., Jing, L., & Chenglong, Z. (2020). Magnesium oil enriched transdermal nanogel of methotrexate for improved arthritic joint mobility, repair, and reduced inflammation. *Journal of*

microencapsulation, *37*(1), 77–90. https://doi.org/10.1080/02652048.2019.1694086.

153. NIH, National Institute of General Medical Sciences (NIGMS). (2013). The biology of fats in the body. *ScienceDaily*. Retrieved July 29, 2020 from www.sciencedaily.com/releases/2013/04/130423102127.htm.
154. Wang, D. D., Li, Y., Chiuve, S. E., Stampfer, M. J., Manson, J. E., Rimm, E. B., Willett, W. C., & Hu, F. B. (2016). Association of Specific Dietary Fats With Total and Cause-Specific Mortality. *JAMA internal medicine*, *176*(8), 1134–1145. https://doi.org/10.1001/jamainternmed.2016.2417.
155. Yngve A. (2009). A Historical Perspective of the Understanding of the Link between Diet and Coronary Heart Disease. *American journal of lifestyle medicine*, *3*(1 Suppl.), 35S–38S. https://doi.org/10.1177/1559827609334887.
156. Esposito, K., Marfella, R., Ciotola, M., Di Palo, C., Giugliano, F., Giugliano, G., D'Armiento, M., D'Andrea, F., & Giugliano, D. (2004). Effect of a Mediterranean-style diet on endothelial dysfunction and markers of vascular inflammation in the metabolic syndrome: a randomized trial. *JAMA*, *292*(12), 1440–1446. https://doi.org/10.1001/jama.292.12.1440.
157. Chrysohoou, C., Panagiotakos, D. B., Pitsavos, C., Das, U. N., & Stefanadis, C. (2004). Adherence to the Mediterranean diet attenuates inflammation and coagulation process in healthy adults: The ATTICA Study. *Journal of the American College of Cardiology*, *44*(1), 152–158. https://doi.org/10.1016/j.jacc.2004.03.039.
158. Matsumoto, Y., Sugioka, Y., Tada, M., Okano, T., Mamoto, K., Inui, K., Habu, D., & Koike, T. (2018). Monounsaturated fatty acids might be key factors in the Mediterranean diet that suppress rheumatoid arthritis disease activity: The TOMORROW study. *Clinical nutrition (Edinburgh, Scotland)*, *37*(2), 675–680. https://doi.org/10.1016/j.clnu.2017.02.011.
159. Lu, B., Driban, J. B., Xu, C., Lapane, K. L., McAlindon, T. E., & Eaton, C. B. (2017). Dietary Fat Intake and Radiographic Progression of Knee Osteoarthritis: Data From the Osteoarthritis Initiative. *Arthritis care & research*, *69*(3), 368–375. https://doi.org/10.1002/acr.22952.
160. Simopoulos A. P. (2008). The importance of the omega-6/omega-3 fatty acid ratio in cardiovascular disease and other chronic diseases. *Experimental biology and medicine (Maywood, N.J.)*, *233*(6), 674–688. https://doi.org/10.3181/0711-MR-311.
161. Ullah, R., Nadeem, M., Khalique, A., Imran, M., Mehmood, S., Javid, A., & Hussain, J. (2016). Nutritional and therapeutic perspectives of Chia (*Salvia hispanica L.*): a review. *Journal of food science and technology*, *53*(4), 1750–1758. https://doi.org/10.1007/s13197-015-1967-0.

162. Domenichiello, A. F., Kitson, A. P., & Bazinet, R. P. (2015). Is docosahexaenoic acid synthesis from α-linolenic acid sufficient to supply the adult brain?. *Progress in lipid research*, *59*, 54–66. https://doi.org/10.1016/j.plipres.2015.04.002.
163. Hill, C., Guarner, F., Reid, G., Gibson, G. R., Merenstein, D. J., Pot, B., Morelli, L., Canani, R. B., Flint, H. J., Salminen, S., Calder, P. C., & Sanders, M. E. (2014). Expert consensus document. The International Scientific Association for Probiotics and Prebiotics consensus statement on the scope and appropriate use of the term probiotic. *Nature reviews. Gastroenterology & hepatology*, *11*(8), 506–514. https://doi.org/10.1038/nrgastro.2014.66.
164. Megan, R. (2019). *Eat Yourself Healthy: An Easy-to-digest Guide to Health and Happiness from the Inside Out*. London: Penguin Life.
165. Valdes A. M, Walter J., Segal E., Spector T.D. (2018). Role of the gut microbiota in nutrition and health, *BMJ 361;k2179*. https://www.bmj.com/content/361/bmj.k2179.
166. Ma, Y., Hébert, J. R., Li, W., Bertone-Johnson, E. R., Olendzki, B., Pagoto, S. L., Tinker, L., Rosal, M. C., Ockene, I. S., Ockene, J. K., Griffith, J. A., & Liu, S. (2008). Association between dietary fiber and markers of systemic inflammation in the Women's Health Initiative Observational Study. *Nutrition (Burbank, Los Angeles County, Calif.)*, *24*(10), 941–949. https://doi.org/10.1016/j.nut.2008.04.005.

References – Chapter 3

1. Kunnumakkara, A. B., Sailo, B. L., Banik, K., Harsha, C., Prasad, S., Gupta, S. C., Bharti, A. C., & Aggarwal, B. B. (2018). Chronic diseases, inflammation, and spices: how are they linked?. *Journal of translational medicine*, *16*(1), 14. https://doi.org/10.1186/s12967-018-1381-2.
2. Macchiochi J (2020), *Immunity: The Science of Staying Well*, London: Thorsons.
3. Kunnumakkara, A. B., Sailo, B. L., Banik, K., Harsha, C., Prasad, S., Gupta, S. C., Bharti, A. C., & Aggarwal, B. B. (2018). Chronic diseases, inflammation, and spices: how are they linked?. *Journal of translational medicine*, *16*(1), 14. https://doi.org/10.1186/s12967-018-1381-2.
4. O'Brien, A., Backman, C. (2010). Chapter 16 - Inflammatory arthritis, *Rheumatology*, 211-233, https://doi.org/10.1016/B978-0-443-06934-5.00016-4.
5. Robinson, W. H., Lepus, C. M., Wang, Q., Raghu, H., Mao, R., Lindstrom, T. M., & Sokolove, J. (2016). Low-grade inflammation as a key mediator of the pathogenesis of osteoarthritis. *Nature reviews. Rheumatology*, *12*(10), 580–592. https://doi.org/10.1038/nrrheum.2016.136.

6. Pahwa, R., Goyal, A., Bansal, P., & Jialal, I. (2020). Chronic Inflammation. In *StatPearls*. StatPearls Publishing. Available from: https://www.ncbi.nlm.nih.gov/books/NBK493173/.
7. Statovci, D., Aguilera, M., MacSharry, J., & Melgar, S. (2017). The Impact of Western Diet and Nutrients on the Microbiota and Immune Response at Mucosal Interfaces. *Frontiers in immunology*, *8*, 838. https://doi.org/10.3389/fimmu.2017.00838.
8. World Health Organization. (2020, April 1). Obesity and overweight 2020. *Fact Sheets*. https://www.who.int/news-room/fact-sheets/detail/obesity-and-overweight.
9. Tan Monique, He Feng J, MacGregor Graham A. (2020). Obesity and covid-19: the role of the food industry, *BMJ, 369,* doi: https://doi.org/10.1136/bmj.m2237.
10. Spector T (2016), *The Diet Myth,* London: Weidenfield & Nicolson. Extracts also available online: https://theconversation.com/your-gut-bacteria-dont-like-junk-food-even-if-you-do-41564.
11. Anderson, S., C., Cryan, J., F., Dinan, T. (2019). *The Psychobiotic Revolution*, Washington:National Geographic Partners, LLC.
12. DiNicolantonio, J. J., & O'Keefe, J. H. (2017). Good Fats versus Bad Fats: A Comparison of Fatty Acids in the Promotion of Insulin Resistance, Inflammation, and Obesity. *Missouri medicine*, *114*(4), 303–307. Accessed via https://www.ncbi.nlm.nih.gov/pmc/articles/PMC6140086/.
13. WWF-UK. (2020, January 17). 8 Things to Know Aout Palm Oil, *Palm Oil Scorecard*. https://www.wwf.org.uk/updates/8-things-know-about-palm-oil#:~:text=Palm%20oil%20has%20been%20and,pygmy%20elephant%20and%20Sumatran%20rhino. (Accessed 29.07.2020).
14. Aro, A., Antoine, J., M., Pizzoferrato, L., Reykdal, O., van Poppel, G. (1998). Trans Fatty Acids in Dairy and Meat Products from 14 European Countries: The TRANSFAIR Study, *Journal of Food Composition and Analysis,* 11(2): 150-160, https://doi.org/10.1006/jfca.1998.0570.
15. Mozaffarian, D., Katan, M. B., Ascherio, A., Stampfer, M. J., & Willett, W. C. (2006). Trans fatty acids and cardiovascular disease. *The New England journal of medicine*, *354*(15), 1601–1613. https://doi.org/10.1056/NEJMra054035.
16. Mozaffarian D. (2006). Trans fatty acids - effects on systemic inflammation and endothelial function. *Atherosclerosis. Supplements*, 7(2), 29–32. https://doi.org/10.1016/j.atherosclerosissup.2006.04.007.
17. Giugliano, D., Ceriello, A., & Esposito, K. (2006). The effects of diet on inflammation: emphasis on the metabolic syndrome. *Journal of the*

American College of Cardiology, *48*(4), 677–685. https://doi.org/10.1016/j.jacc.2006.03.052.

18. Esposito, K., Nappo, F., Marfella, R., Giugliano, G., Giugliano, F., Ciotola, M., Quagliaro, L., Ceriello, A., & Giugliano, D. (2002). Inflammatory cytokine concentrations are acutely increased by hyperglycemia in humans: role of oxidative stress. *Circulation*, *106*(16), 2067–2072. https://doi.org/10.1161/01.cir.0000034509.14906.ae.
19. Della Corte, K. W., Perrar, I., Penczynski, K. J., Schwingshackl, L., Herder, C., & Buyken, A. E. (2018). Effect of Dietary Sugar Intake on Biomarkers of Subclinical Inflammation: A Systematic Review and Meta-Analysis of Intervention Studies. *Nutrients*, *10*(5), 606. https://doi.org/10.3390/nu10050606.
20. Westover, A. N., & Marangell, L. B. (2002). A cross-national relationship between sugar consumption and major depression?. *Depression and anxiety*, *16*(3), 118–120. https://doi.org/10.1002/da.10054.
21. Stokstad, E. (2015). Humans have been using bees for at least 9000 years. *Science: Plants & Animals*. doi:10.1126/science.aad7421.
22. Badolato, M., Carullo, G., Cione, E., Aiello, F., & Caroleo, M. C. (2017). From the hive: Honey, a novel weapon against cancer. *European journal of medicinal chemistry*, *142*, 290–299. https://doi.org/10.1016/j.ejmech.2017.07.064.
23. Sanz, M. L., Polemis, N., Morales, V., Corzo, N., Drakoularakou, A., Gibson, G. R., & Rastall, R. A. (2005). In vitro investigation into the potential prebiotic activity of honey oligosaccharides. Journal of agricultural and food chemistry, 53(8), 2914–2921. https://doi.org/10.1021/jf0500684.
24. Sigaux, J., Semerano, L., Favre, G., Bessis, N., & Boissier, M. C. (2018). Salt, inflammatory joint disease, and autoimmunity. *Joint bone spine*, *85*(4), 411–416. https://doi.org/10.1016/j.jbspin.2017.06.003.
25. Cani, P. D., & Everard, A. (2015). Keeping gut lining at bay: impact of emulsifiers. *Trends in endocrinology and metabolism: TEM*, *26*(6), 273–274. https://doi.org/10.1016/j.tem.2015.03.009.
26. Bartolotto C. (2015). Does Consuming Sugar and Artificial Sweeteners Change Taste Preferences?. *The Permanente journal*, 19(3), 81–84. https://doi.org/10.7812/TPP/14-229.
27. Suez, J., Koram, T., Zilberman-Schapira, G., Segal, E., Elinav, E. (2015). Non-caloric artificial sweeteners and the microbiome: findings and challenges. Gut Microbes, 6(2), 149-155. doi: 10.1080/19490976.2015.1017700.
28. Wu, G. D., Chen, J., Hoffmann, C., Bittinger, K., Chen, Y. Y., Keilbaugh, S. A., Bewtra, M., Knights, D., Walters, W. A., Knight, R., Sinha, R., Gilroy, E., Gupta, K., Baldassano, R., Nessel, L., Li, H., Bushman, F. D., & Lewis, J. D. (2011). Linking long-term dietary patterns with gut microbial

enterotypes. *Science (New York, N.Y.), 334*(6052), 105–108. https://doi.org/10.1126/science.1208344.

29. Abou-Donia, M. B., El-Masry, E. M., Abdel-Rahman, A. A., McLendon, R. E., & Schiffman, S. S. (2008). Splenda alters gut microflora and increases intestinal p-glycoprotein and cytochrome p-450 in male rats. *Journal of toxicology and environmental health. Part A*, *71*(21), 1415–1429. https://doi.org/10.1080/15287390802328630.
30. Case Western Reserve University. (2018, March 15). Artificial sweetener could intensify symptoms in those with Crohn's disease: Promotes 'bad' bacteria and intestinal inflammation; findings may guide dietary habits in human patients. *ScienceDaily.* Retrieved August 2, 2020 from www.sciencedaily.com/releases/2018/03/180315155411.htm.
31. Bian, X., Chi, L., Gao, B., Tu, P., Ru, H., & Lu, K. (2017). Gut Microbiome Response to Sucralose and Its Potential Role in Inducing Liver Inflammation in Mice. Frontiers in physiology, 8, 487. https://doi.org/10.3389/fphys.2017.00487.
32. Gerasimidis, K., Bryden, K., Chen, X., Papachristou, E., Verney, A., Roig, M., Hansen, R., Nichols, B., Papadopoulou, R., & Parrett, A. (2020). The impact of food additives, artificial sweeteners and domestic hygiene products on the human gut microbiome and its fibre fermentation capacity. *European journal of nutrition*, *59*(7), 3213–3230. https://doi.org/10.1007/s00394-019-02161-8.
33. Name of strain of bacteria: *Mycobacterium avium subspecies paratuberculosis.*
34. Fasano A. (2012). Zonulin, regulation of tight junctions, and autoimmune diseases. *Annals of the New York Academy of Sciences*, *1258*(1), 25–33. https://doi.org/10.1111/j.1749-6632.2012.06538.x.
35. Muthuri, S. G., Zhang, W., Maciewicz, R. A., Muir, K., & Doherty, M. (2015). Beer and wine consumption and risk of knee or hip osteoarthritis: a case control study. *Arthritis research & therapy*, *17*(1), 23. https://doi.org/10.1186/s13075-015-0534-4.
36. Shield, K. D., Parry, C., & Rehm, J. (2013). Chronic diseases and conditions related to alcohol use. *Alcohol research: current reviews*, *35*(2), 155–173.
37. NHS UK. (2018). What are the health risks of smoking?, *NHS: Common Health Questions, Lifestyle.* https://www.nhs.uk/common-health-questions/lifestyle/what-are-the-health-risks-of-smoking/#:~:text=Every%20year%20around%2078%2C000%20people,term%20damage%20to%20your%20health. Accessed 12.08.2020.
38. Pezzolo, E., & Naldi, L. (2019). The relationship between smoking, psoriasis and psoriatic arthritis. *Expert review of clinical immunology*, *15*(1), 41–48. https://doi.org/10.1080/1744666X.2019.1543591.

39. Lee, J., Taneja, V., & Vassallo, R. (2012). Cigarette smoking and inflammation: cellular and molecular mechanisms. *Journal of dental research*, *91*(2), 142–149. https://doi.org/10.1177/0022034511421200.
40. Adams, S. (2010, December 14). Smoking 'causes a third of severe rheumatoid arthritis cases', *The Telegraph*. https://www.telegraph.co.uk/news/health/news/8198868/Smoking-causes-a-third-of-severe-rheumatoid-arthritis-cases.html. Accessed 13.08.2020.
41. Di Giuseppe, D., Discacciati, A., Orsini, N., & Wolk, A. (2014). Cigarette smoking and risk of rheumatoid arthritis: a dose-response meta-analysis. *Arthritis research & therapy*, *16*(2), R61. https://doi.org/10.1186/ar4498.
42. Hedström, A. K., Stawiarz, L., Klareskog, L., & Alfredsson, L. (2018). Smoking and susceptibility to rheumatoid arthritis in a Swedish population-based case-control study. *European journal of epidemiology*, *33*(4), 415–423. https://doi.org/10.1007/s10654-018-0360-5.
43. Aparicio-Soto, M., Sánchez-Hidalgo, M., Rosillo, M. Á., Castejón, M. L., & Alarcón-de-la-Lastra, C. (2016). Extra virgin olive oil: a key functional food for prevention of immune-inflammatory diseases. *Food & function*, 7(11), 4492–4505. https://doi.org/10.1039/c6fo01094f.
44. Sköldstam, L., Hagfors, L., & Johansson, G. (2003). An experimental study of a Mediterranean diet intervention for patients with rheumatoid arthritis. *Annals of the rheumatic diseases*, *62*(3), 208–214. https://doi.org/10.1136/ard.62.3.208.

References – Chapter 4

1. Loreto A. Muñoz, Angel Cobos, Olga Diaz & José Miguel Aguilera (2013) Chia Seed (*Salvia hispanica*): An Ancient Grain and a New Functional Food, Food Reviews International, 29:4, 394-408, DOI: 10.1080/87559129.2013.818014
2. Koner, S., Pratyasha Dash, P., Priya, V., Rajeswari, D., 15 - Natural and Artificial Beverages: Exploring the Pros and Cons, *Natural Beverages*, 427-445, https://doi.org/10.1016/B978-0-12-816689-5.00015-8.
3. Suri, S., Passi, J. S., Goyat, J. (2016). Chia Seed (*Salvia Hispanica L.*) – A New Age Functional Food. *4th International Conference on Recent Innovations in Science Engineering and Management*. https://www.ijates.com/images/short_pdf/1459080855_695I.pdf.
4. Pathak, S., Kesavan, P., Banerjee, A., Banerjee, A., Sagdicoglu G.,C., Bissi, L., Marotta, F., (2018). Chapter 25 - Metabolism of Dietary Polyphenols by Human Gut Microbiota and Their Health Benefits, *Polyphenols: Mechanisms of Action in Human Health and Disease (Second Edition)*, 347-359,

https://doi.org/10.1016/B978-0-12-813006-3.00025-8.

5. Lockwood, G.B. (2009). Chapter 32 - The plant nutraceuticals, *Trease and Evans' Pharmacognosy (Sixteenth Edition)*, 459-470, https://doi.org/10.1016/B978-0-7020-2933-2.00032-0.
6. Ledbetter, C. (2017). It Turns Out You're Eating Flaxseeds All Wrong. *Huffington Post UK*. https://www.huffingtonpost.co.uk/entry/it-turns-out-youre-eating-flaxseeds-all-wrong_n_59aedc61e4b0b5e531014f35 (Accessed 06.07.2020).
7. Dodd, F. L., Kennedy, D. O., Riby, L. M., & Haskell-Ramsay, C. F. (2015). A double-blind, placebo-controlled study evaluating the effects of caffeine and L-theanine both alone and in combination on cerebral blood flow, cognition and mood. *Psychopharmacology*, *232*(14), 2563–2576. https://doi.org/10.1007/s00213-015-3895-0.
8. Nobre, A. C., Rao, A., & Owen, G. N. (2008). L-theanine, a natural constituent in tea, and its effect on mental state. *Asia Pacific journal of clinical nutrition*, *17 Suppl 1*, 167–168.
9. Dietz, C., Dekker, M., & Piqueras-Fiszman, B. (2017). An intervention study on the effect of matcha tea, in drink and snack bar formats, on mood and cognitive performance. *Food research international (Ottawa, Ont.)*, *99*(Pt 1), 72–83. https://doi.org/10.1016/j.foodres.2017.05.002.
10. Shubrook, N. (2018). The Health Benefits of Maca Powder. *BBC Good Food*. https://www.bbcgoodfood.com/howto/guide/health-benefits-maca-powder.
11. di Giuseppe, R., Di Castelnuovo, A., Centritto, F., Zito, F., De Curtis, A., Costanzo, S., Vohnout, B., Sieri, S., Krogh, V., Donati, M. B., de Gaetano, G., & Iacoviello, L. (2008). Regular consumption of dark chocolate is associated with low serum concentrations of C-reactive protein in a healthy Italian population. *The Journal of nutrition*, *138*(10), 1939–1945. https://doi.org/10.1093/jn/138.10.1939.
12. Stohs, S. J., & Hartman, M. J. (2015). Review of the Safety and Efficacy of *Moringa oleifera*. *Phytotherapy research: PTR*, *29*(6), 796–804. https://doi.org/10.1002/ptr.5325.
13. Škrabanja, V., Kreft, I. (2016). Chapter thirteen - Nutritional Value of Buckwheat Proteins and Starch, Molecular Breeding and Nutritional Aspects of Buckwheat, 169-176, https://doi.org/10.1016/B978-0-12-803692-1.00013-4.
14. Zieliński, H., & Kozłowska, H. (2000). Antioxidant activity and total phenolics in selected cereal grains and their different morphological fractions. *Journal of agricultural and food chemistry*, *48*(6), 2008–2016. https://doi.org/10.1021/jf990619o.
15. Ahmed, A., Khalid, N., Ahmad, A., Abbasi, N., Latif, M., & Randhawa, M. (2014). Phytochemicals and biofunctional properties of buckwheat: A

review. *The Journal of Agricultural Science, 152(3)*, 349-369. doi:10.1017/S0021859613000166.

16. Jong, S. C., & Birmingham, J. M. (1993). Medicinal and therapeutic value of the shiitake mushroom. *Advances in applied microbiology*, *39*, 153–184. https://doi.org/10.1016/s0065-2164(08)70595-1.
17. Reis, F. S., Barros, L., Martins, A., & Ferreira, I. C. (2012). Chemical composition and nutritional value of the most widely appreciated cultivated mushrooms: an inter-species comparative study. *Food and chemical toxicology : an international journal published for the British Industrial Biological Research Association*, *50*(2), 191–197. https://doi.org/10.1016/j.fct.2011.10.056.
18. Jong, S. C., & Birmingham, J. M. (1993). Medicinal and therapeutic value of the shiitake mushroom. *Advances in applied microbiology*, 39, 153–184. https://doi.org/10.1016/s0065-2164(08)70595-1.
19. Dai, X., Stanilka, J. M., Rowe, C. A., Esteves, E. A., Nieves, C., Jr, Spaiser, S. J., Christman, M. C., Langkamp-Henken, B., & Percival, S. S. (2015). Consuming *Lentinula edodes* (Shiitake) Mushrooms Daily Improves Human Immunity: A Randomized Dietary Intervention in Healthy Young Adults. *Journal of the American College of Nutrition*, *34*(6), 478–487. https://doi.org/10.1080/07315724.2014.950391.
20. Yang, Cheng-Hong & Chang, Fang-Rong & Chang, Hsueh-Wei & Wang, Shao-Ming & Hsieh, Ming-Che & Chuang, Li-Yeh. (2012). Investigation of the antioxidant activity of *Illicium verum* extracts. *Journal of Medicinal Plants Research*. 6.
21. Callaway, J.C. (2004). Hempseed as a nutritional resource: An overview. *Euphytica* 140, 65–72. https://doi.org/10.1007/s10681-004-4811-6.
22. Kuligowski, M., Jasińska-Kuligowska, I., & Nowak, J. (2013). Evaluation of bean and soy tempeh influence on intestinal bacteria and estimation of antibacterial properties of bean tempeh. *Polish journal of microbiology*, *62*(2), 189–194.
23. Nuraida, L., (2015). A review: Health promoting lactic acid bacteria in traditional Indonesian fermented foods, *Food Science and Human Wellness*, 4(2): 47-55, https://doi.org/10.1016/j.fshw.2015.06.001.
24. Nikodinovic-Runic, J., Guzik, M., Kenny, S. T., Babu, R., Werker, A., & O Connor, K. E. (2013). Carbon-rich wastes as feedstocks for biodegradable polymer (polyhydroxyalkanoate) production using bacteria. *Advances in applied microbiology*, *84*, 139–200. https://doi.org/10.1016/B978-0-12-407673-0.00004-7.
25. Urban Dictionary. (2017, April 12). *Definition: Vegan Crack*. https://www.urbandictionary.com/define.php?term=vegan+crack.

26. Navruz-Varli, S., Sanlier, N. (2016). Nutritional and health benefits of quinoa (*Chenopodium quinoa* Willd.), *Journal of Cereal Science*, 69: 371-376. https://doi.org/10.1016/j.jcs.2016.05.004.
27. Farnworth, Edward. (2005). Kefir - A complex probiotic. *Food Science & Technology Bulletin: Functional Foods*. 2. 1-17. 10.1616/1476-2137.13938.
28. Prado, M. R., Blandón, L. M., Vandenberghe, L. P., Rodrigues, C., Castro, G. R., Thomaz-Soccol, V., & Soccol, C. R. (2015). Milk kefir: composition, microbial cultures, biological activities, and related products. *Frontiers in microbiology*, 6, 1177. https://doi.org/10.3389/fmicb.2015.01177.
29. Golowczyc, M. A., Mobili, P., Garrote, G. L., Abraham, A. G., & De Antoni, G. L. (2007). Protective action of Lactobacillus kefir carrying S-layer protein against Salmonella enterica serovar Enteritidis. *International journal of food microbiology*, *118*(3), 264–273. https://doi.org/10.1016/j.ijfoodmicro.2007.07.042.
30. de Oliveira Leite, A. M., Miguel, M. A., Peixoto, R. S., Rosado, A. S., Silva, J. T., & Paschoalin, V. M. (2013). Microbiological, technological and therapeutic properties of kefir: a natural probiotic beverage. *Brazilian journal of microbiology : [publication of the Brazilian Society for Microbiology]*, 44(2), 341–349. https://doi.org/10.1590/S1517-83822013000200001.

References – Chapter 5

1. Cerhan, J. R., Saag, K. G., Merlino, L. A., Mikuls, T. R., & Criswell, L. A. (2003). Antioxidant micronutrients and risk of rheumatoid arthritis in a cohort of older women. *American journal of epidemiology*, *157*(4), 345–354. https://doi.org/10.1093/aje/kwf205.

References – Chapter 6

1. Omoigui S. (2007). The biochemical origin of pain: the origin of all pain is inflammation and the inflammatory response. Part 2 of 3 - inflammatory profile of pain syndromes. *Medical hypotheses*, 69(6), 1169–1178. https://doi.org/10.1016/j.mehy.2007.06.033.
2. Zhang, J. M., & An, J. (2007). Cytokines, inflammation, and pain. *International anesthesiology clinics*, 45(2), 27–37. https://doi.org/10.1097/AIA.0b013e318034194e.
3. NHS Digital. (2018, December 4). Health Survey for England 2017 [NS]. *Publication, Part of Health Survey for England*. https://digital.nhs.uk/data-and-information/publications/statistical/health-survey-for-england/2017.
4. Versus Arthritis (2019). 'The State of Musculoskeletal Health 2019.' *versusarthritis.org*. Retrieved from: https://www.versusarthritis.org/media/14594/state-of-musculoskeletal-health-2019.pdf.

5. Engel G. L. (1977). The need for a new medical model: a challenge for biomedicine. Science (New York, N.Y.), 196(4286), 129–136. https://doi.org/10.1126/science.847460.
6. Felitti, V. J., Anda, R. F., Nordenberg, D., Williamson, D. F., Spitz, A. M., Edwards, V., Koss, M. P., & Marks, J. S. (1998). Relationship of childhood abuse and household dysfunction to many of the leading causes of death in adults. The Adverse Childhood Experiences (ACE) Study. American journal of preventive medicine, 14(4), 245–258. https://doi.org/10.1016/s0749-3797(98)00017-8.
7. Potter, N. (2019). *The Meaning of Pain*. London: Short Books.
8. Hassett, A. L., & Clauw, D. J. (2010). The role of stress in rheumatic diseases. Arthritis research & therapy, 12(3), 123. https://doi.org/10.1186/ar3024.
9. Breit, S., Kupferberg, A., Rogler, G., & Hasler, G. (2018). Vagus Nerve as Modulator of the Brain-Gut Axis in Psychiatric and Inflammatory Disorders. *Frontiers in psychiatry*, *9*, 44. https://doi.org/10.3389/fpsyt.2018.00044.
10. Goverse, G., Stakenborg, M., & Matteoli, G. (2016). The intestinal cholinergic anti-inflammatory pathway. *The Journal of physiology*, *594*(20), 5771–5780. https://doi.org/10.1113/JP271537.
11. George, M. S., Ward, H. E., Jr, Ninan, P. T., Pollack, M., Nahas, Z., Anderson, B., Kose, S., Howland, R. H., Goodman, W. K., & Ballenger, J. C. (2008). A pilot study of vagus nerve stimulation (VNS) for treatment-resistant anxiety disorders. *Brain stimulation*, *1*(2), 112–121.
12. Rod K. (2015). Observing the Effects of Mindfulness-Based Meditation on Anxiety and Depression in Chronic Pain Patients. *Psychiatria Danubina*, *27 Suppl 1*, S209–S211.
13. Koopman, F. A., Chavan, S. S., Miljko, S., Grazio, S., Sokolovic, S., Schuurman, P. R., Mehta, A. D., Levine, Y. A., Faltys, M., Zitnik, R., Tracey, K. J., & Tak, P. P. (2016). Vagus nerve stimulation inhibits cytokine production and attenuates disease severity in rheumatoid arthritis. Proceedings of the National Academy of Sciences of the United States of America, 113(29), 8284–8289. https://doi.org/10.1073/pnas.1605635113.
14. Hong, J. I., Park, I. Y., & Kim, H. A. (2020). Understanding the Molecular Mechanisms Underlying the Pathogenesis of Arthritis Pain Using Animal Models. International journal of molecular sciences, 21(2), 533. https://doi.org/10.3390/ijms21020533.
15. Woolf C. J. (2011). Central sensitization: implications for the diagnosis and treatment of pain. Pain, 152(3 Suppl), S2–S15. https://doi.org/10.1016/j.pain.2010.09.030.
16. Rifbjerg-Madsen, S., Christensen, A. W., Christensen, R., Hetland, M. L., Bliddal, H., Kristensen, L. E., Danneskiold-Samsøe, B., & Amris, K.

(2017). Pain and pain mechanisms in patients with inflammatory arthritis: A Danish nationwide cross-sectional DANBIO registry survey. PloS one, 12(7), e0180014. https://doi.org/10.1371/journal.pone.0180014.

17. de Baaij, J. H., Hoenderop, J. G., & Bindels, R. J. (2015). Magnesium in man: implications for health and disease. Physiological reviews, 95(1), 1–46. https://doi.org/10.1152/physrev.00012.2014.

18. Peuhkuri, K., Sihvola, N., & Korpela, R. (2012). Dietary factors and fluctuating levels of melatonin. Food & nutrition research, 56, 10.3402/fnr.v56i0.17252. https://doi.org/10.3402/fnr.v56i0.17252.

19. Gröber, U., Werner, T., Vormann, J., & Kisters, K. (2017). Myth or Reality-Transdermal Magnesium?. Nutrients, 9(8), 813. https://doi.org/10.3390/nu9080813.

20. Hill, K. P., Palastro, M. D., Johnson, B., & Ditre, J. W. (2017). Cannabis and Pain: A Clinical Review. Cannabis and cannabinoid research, 2(1), 96–104. https://doi.org/10.1089/can.2017.0017.

21. Russo E. B. (2007). History of cannabis and its preparations in saga, science, and sobriquet. Chemistry & biodiversity, 4(8), 1614–1648. https://doi.org/10.1002/cbdv.200790144.

22. The Rt Hon Sajid Javid MP. (2018, October 11). Government announces that medicinal cannabis is legal. *Gov.UK, Home Office*. https://www.gov.uk/government/news/government-announces-that-medicinal-cannabis-is-legal.

23. Morales P., Hurst D.P., Reggio P.H. (2017) Molecular Targets of the Phytocannabinoids: A Complex Picture. In: Kinghorn A., Falk H., Gibbons S., Kobayashi J. (eds) *Phytocannabinoids. Progress in the Chemistry of Organic Natural Products*, vol 103. Springer, Cham. https://doi.org/10.1007/978-3-319-45541-9_4.

24. Gordon, D. (2020). *The CBD Bible: Cannabis and the Wellness Revolution That Will Change Your Life*. London: Orion Spring.

25. National Academies of Sciences, Engineering, and Medicine, Health and Medicine Division, Board on Population Health and Public Health Practice, & Committee on the Health Effects of Marijuana: An Evidence Review and Research Agenda. (2017). The Health Effects of Cannabis and Cannabinoids: The Current State of Evidence and Recommendations for Research. National Academies Press (US). doi: 10.17226/24625.

26. Hammell, D. C., Zhang, L. P., Ma, F., Abshire, S. M., McIlwrath, S. L., Stinchcomb, A. L., & Westlund, K. N. (2016). Transdermal cannabidiol reduces inflammation and pain-related behaviours in a rat model of arthritis. *European Journal of Pain (London, England)*, *20*(6), 936–948. https://doi.org/10.1002/ejp.818.

27. Malfait, A. M., Gallily, R., Sumariwalla, P. F., Malik, A. S., Andreakos, E., Mechoulam, R., & Feldmann, M. (2000). The nonpsychoactive cannabis constituent cannabidiol is an oral anti-arthritic therapeutic in murine collagen-induced arthritis. *Proceedings of the National Academy of Sciences of the United States of America*, 97(17), 9561–9566. https://doi.org/10.1073/pnas.160105897.
28. Fitzcharles, M. A., Baerwald, C., Ablin, J., & Häuser, W. (2016). Efficacy, tolerability and safety of cannabinoids in chronic pain associated with rheumatic diseases (fibromyalgia syndrome, back pain, osteoarthritis, rheumatoid arthritis): A systematic review of randomized controlled trials. *Schmerz (Berlin, Germany)*, *30*(1), 47–61. https://doi.org/10.1007/s00482-015-0084-3.
29. Pushpangadan, P., Tewari, S.K. (2006). 28 – Peppermint, *Woodhead Publishing Series in Food Science, Technology and Nutrition, Handbook of Herbs and Spices,* 3(28): 460-481, https://doi.org/10.1533/9781845691717.3.460.
30. Memariani, Z., Gorji, N., Moeini, R., Hosein Farzaei, M. (2020). Chapter Two - Traditional uses, Phytonutrients in Food, 23-66, https://doi.org/10.1016/B978-0-12-815354-3.00004-6.
31. Taneja, S.C., Chandra, S., (2012). 20 - Mint, *Woodhead Publishing Series in Food Science, Technology and Nutrition, Handbook of Herbs and Spices (Second Edition),* 366-387, https://doi.org/10.1533/9780857095671.366.
32. Schmidt, E., Bail, S., Buchbauer, G., Stoilova, I., Atanasova, T., Stoyanova, A., Krastanov, A., & Jirovetz, L. (2009). Chemical composition, olfactory evaluation and antioxidant effects of essential oil from *Mentha x piperita*. Natural product communications, 4(8), 1107–1112.
33. Eccles, R. (1994), Menthol and Related Cooling Compounds. *Journal of Pharmacy and Pharmacology,* 46: 618-630. doi:10.1111/j.2042-7158.1994.tb03871.x
34. Riachi, L. G., De Maria, C. A.B. (2015). Peppermint antioxidants revisited, Food Chemistry,176: 72-81, https://doi.org/10.1016/j.foodchem.2014.12.028.
35. Surjushe, A., Vasani, R., & Saple, D. G. (2008). Aloe vera: a short review. Indian journal of dermatology, 53(4), 163–166. https://doi.org/10.4103/0019-5154.44785.
36. Salehi, B., Albayrak, S., Antolak, H., Kręgiel, D., Pawlikowska, E., Sharifi-Rad, M., Uprety, Y., Tsouh Fokou, P. V., Yousef, Z., Amiruddin Zakaria, Z., Varoni, E. M., Sharopov, F., Martins, N., Iriti, M., & Sharifi-Rad, J. (2018). Aloe Genus Plants: From Farm to Food Applications and Phytopharmacotherapy. International journal of molecular sciences, 19(9), 2843. https://doi.org/10.3390/ijms19092843.

37. Davis, R. H., Rosenthal, K. Y., Cesario, L. R., & Rouw, G. A. (1989). Processed Aloe vera administered topically inhibits inflammation. Journal of the American Podiatric Medical Association, 79(8), 395–397. https://doi.org/10.7547/87507315-79-8-395.
38. Bhardwaj, A., Misra, K. (2018). Chapter 11 - Homeopathic Remedies, Management of High Altitude Pathophysiology, 217-229, https://doi.org/10.1016/B978-0-12-813999-8.00011-2.
39. Salehi, B., Albayrak, S., Antolak, H., Kręgiel, D., Pawlikowska, E., Sharifi-Rad, M., Uprety, Y., Tsouh Fokou, P. V., Yousef, Z., Amiruddin Zakaria, Z., Varoni, E. M., Sharopov, F., Martins, N., Iriti, M., & Sharifi-Rad, J. (2018). Aloe Genus Plants: From Farm to Food Applications and Phytopharmacotherapy. International journal of molecular sciences, 19(9), 2843. https://doi.org/10.3390/ijms19092843.
40. Yoo, E. A., Kim, S. D., Lee, W. M., Park, H. J., Kim, S. K., Cho, J. Y., Min, W., & Rhee, M. H. (2008). Evaluation of antioxidant, antinociceptive, and anti-inflammatory activities of ethanol extracts from *Aloe saponaria Haw. Phytotherapy research: PTR*, 22(10), 1389–1395. https://doi.org/10.1002/ptr.2514.
41. Vandana, K. R., Yalavarthi, P. R., Sundaresan, C. R., Sriramaneni, R. N., & Vadlamudi, H. C. (2014). In-vitro assessment and pharmacodynamics of nimesulide incorporated Aloe vera transemulgel. *Current drug discovery technologies*, 11(2), 162–167. https://doi.org/10.2174/1570163810666131202233721.
42. Surjushe, A., Vasani, R., & Saple, D. G. (2008). Aloe vera: a short review. *Indian journal of dermatology*, 53(4), 163–166. https://doi.org/10.4103/0019-5154.44785.
43. Nejatzadeh-Barandozi F. (2013). Antibacterial activities and antioxidant capacity of Aloe vera. Organic and medicinal chemistry letters, 3(1), 5. https://doi.org/10.1186/2191-2858-3-5.
44. Tovar, R.T., Petzel, R, M. (2009). Herbal toxicity. *Disease-a-month*, 55(10): 592-641. https://doi.org/10.1016/j.disamonth.2009.05.001.
45. Kline, D., Ritruthai, V., Babajanian, S., Gao, Q., Ingle, P., Chang, P., Swanson, G. (2017). Quantitative Analysis of Aloins and Aloin-Emodin in Aloe Vera Raw Materials and Finished Products Using High-Performance Liquid Chromatography: Single-Laboratory Validation, First Action 2016.09, *Journal of AOAC INTERNATIONAL*, 100(3):661–670, https://doi.org/10.5740/jaoacint.16-0387.
46. Hamed, M., Kalita, D., Bartolo, M. E., & Jayanty, S. S. (2019). Capsaicinoids, Polyphenols and Antioxidant Activities of *Capsicum annuum*: Comparative Study of the Effect of Ripening Stage and Cooking Methods.

Antioxidants (Basel, Switzerland), 8(9), 364. https://doi.org/10.3390/antiox8090364.

47. Zhang, W. Y., & Li Wan Po, A. (1994). The effectiveness of topically applied capsaicin. A meta-analysis. *European journal of clinical pharmacology*, 46(6), 517–522. https://doi.org/10.1007/BF00196108.
48. Berman, B., Lewith, G., Manheimer, E., Bishop, F., L., D'Adamo, C. (2015). 48A - Complementary and alternative medicine, *Rheumatology (Sixth Edition):* 382-389, https://doi.org/10.1016/B978-0-323-09138-1.00048-6.
49. Binsi, P.K., Zynudheen, A.A. (2019). 4 - Functional and Nutraceutical Ingredients, *Marine Resources, Value-Added Ingredients and Enrichments of Beverages,* 101-171, https://doi.org/10.1016/B978-0-12-816687-1.00004-7.
50. Kongtharvonskul, J., Anothaisintawee, T., McEvoy, M., Attia, J., Woratanarat, P., & Thakkinstian, A. (2015). Efficacy and safety of glucosamine, diacerein, and NSAIDs in osteoarthritis knee: a systematic review and network meta-analysis. *European journal of medical research*, *20*(1), 24. https://doi.org/10.1186/s40001-015-0115-7.
51. Zeng, C., Wei, J., Li, H., Wang, Y. L., Xie, D. X., Yang, T., Gao, S. G., Li, Y. S., Luo, W., & Lei, G. H. (2015). Effectiveness and safety of Glucosamine, chondroitin, the two in combination, or celecoxib in the treatment of osteoarthritis of the knee. *Scientific reports*, *5*, 16827. https://doi.org/10.1038/srep16827.
52. Wu, D., Huang, Y., Gu, Y., & Fan, W. (2013). Efficacies of different preparations of glucosamine for the treatment of osteoarthritis: a meta-analysis of randomised, double-blind, placebo-controlled trials. *International journal of clinical practice*, *67*(6), 585–594. https://doi.org/10.1111/ijcp.12115.
53. Wandel, S., Jüni, P., Tendal, B., Nüesch, E., Villiger, P. M., Welton, N. J., Reichenbach, S., & Trelle, S. (2010). Effects of glucosamine, chondroitin, or placebo in patients with osteoarthritis of hip or knee: network meta-analysis. *BMJ (Clinical research ed.)*, *341*, c4675. https://doi.org/10.1136/bmj.c4675.
54. Vriens, J., Nilius, B., & Voets, T. (2014). Peripheral thermosensation in mammals. Nature reviews. Neuroscience, 15(9), 573–589. https://doi.org/10.1038/nrn3784.
55. McDougall J. J. (2006). Arthritis and pain. Neurogenic origin of joint pain. Arthritis research & therapy, 8(6), 220. https://doi.org/10.1186/ar2069.
56. Venkatachalam, K., & Montell, C. (2007). TRP channels. Annual review of biochemistry, 76, 387–417. https://doi.org/10.1146/annurev.biochem.75.103004.142819.
57. National Institure for Health and Care Excellence. (2018, July 11). Rheumatoid arthritis in adults: management. *NICE guideline [NG100]*. https://

www.nice.org.uk/guidance/ng100/chapter/Recommendations#symptom-control.

58. NHS UK. (2019, August 19). Treatment and support - Osteoarthritis. *NHS UK Health A to Z.* https://www.nhs.uk/conditions/osteoarthritis/treatment/.

59. Osiri M, Welch V, Brosseau L et al. (2003) Transcutaneous Electrical Nerve Stimulation for Knee Osteoarthritis. *The Cochrane Library, Issue 3.* Update Software, Oxford.

60. DeDomenico G. (1987). New dimensions in interferential therapy. *A theoretical and clinical guide.* Linfield: Reid Medical.

61. Shimoura, K., Iijima, H., Suzuki, Y., & Aoyama, T. (2019). Immediate Effects of Transcutaneous Electrical Nerve Stimulation on Pain and Physical Performance in Individuals With Preradiographic Knee Osteoarthritis: A Randomized Controlled Trial. Archives of physical medicine and rehabilitation, 100(2), 300–306.e1. https://doi.org/10.1016/j.apmr.2018.08.189.

62. Brosseau, L., Judd, M. G., Marchand, S., Robinson, V. A., Tugwell, P., Wells, G., & Yonge, K. (2003). Transcutaneous electrical nerve stimulation (TENS) for the treatment of rheumatoid arthritis in the hand. *The Cochrane database of systematic reviews*, (3), CD004377. https://doi.org/10.1002/14651858.CD004377.

63. Johnson, M., & Martinson, M. (2007). Efficacy of electrical nerve stimulation for chronic musculoskeletal pain: a meta-analysis of randomized controlled trials. *Pain, 130*(1-2), 157–165. https://doi.org/10.1016/j.pain.2007.02.007.

64. National Center for Complementary and Integrative Health. (2016, January). Acupuncture: In Depth. *NCCIH: Health Information.* https://www.nccih.nih.gov/health/acupuncture-in-depth.

65. Shabert, J., K. (2004). Complementary and Alternative Medicine, *Encyclopedia of Gastroenterology,* 476-482, https://doi.org/10.1016/B0-12-386860-2/00021-6.

66. Perlman, A. I., Sabina, A., Williams, A. L., Njike, V. Y., & Katz, D. L. (2006). Massage therapy for osteoarthritis of the knee: a randomized controlled trial. *Archives of internal medicine*, *166*(22), 2533–2538. https://doi.org/10.1001/archinte.166.22.2533.

67. Perlman, A. I., Ali, A., Njike, V. Y., Hom, D., Davidi, A., Gould-Fogerite, S., Milak, C., & Katz, D. L. (2012). Massage therapy for osteoarthritis of the knee: a randomized dose-finding trial. PloS one, 7(2), e30248. https://doi.org/10.1371/journal.pone.0030248.

68. Field, T., Hernandez-Reif, M., Seligman, S., Krasnegor, J., Sunshine, W., Rivas-Chacon, R., Schanberg, S., & Kuhn, C. (1997). Juvenile rheumatoid

arthritis: benefits from massage therapy. *Journal of pediatric psychology*, 22(5), 607–617. https://doi.org/10.1093/jpepsy/22.5.607.

69. Ghavami, H., Shamsi, S. A., Abdollahpoor, B., Radfar, M., & Khalkhali, H. R. (2019). Impact of hot stone massage therapy on sleep quality in patients on maintenance hemodialysis: A randomized controlled trial. *Journal of research in medical sciences : the official journal of Isfahan University of Medical Sciences*, *24*, 71. https://doi.org/10.4103/jrms.JRMS_734_18.
70. Robinson, N., Lorenc, A., & Liao, X. (2011). The evidence for Shiatsu: a systematic review of Shiatsu and acupressure. BMC complementary and alternative medicine, 11, 88. https://doi.org/10.1186/1472-6882-11-88.
71. Withington BT. (1928). Hippocrates, with an English translation. *Cambridge, MA, Harvard University Press.*
72. Palmer DD. (1910). *The chiropractor's adjustor*. Portland: Portland Printing House.
73. World Health Organization. (2005). World Health Guidelines on basic training and safety in Chiropractic. Switzerland: WHO Press.
74. https://scholar.google.com/scholar_lookup?title=World+Health+Guidelines+on+basic+training+and+safety+in+Chiropractic&publication_year=2005&.
75. Salehi, A., Hashemi, N., Imanieh, M. H., & Saber, M. (2015). Chiropractic: Is it Efficient in Treatment of Diseases? Review of Systematic Reviews. *International journal of community based nursing and midwifery*, *3*(4), 244–254.
76. Judith E. Deutsch. (2018). Chapter 18 - Manipulative and Body-Based Therapies, *Complementary Therapies for Physical Therapy,* 249-263, https://doi.org/10.1016/B978-072160111-3.50024-5.
77. The Chartered Society of Physiotherapy (CSP). (2018, March 14). What is physiotherapy? *CSP: Careers & jobs, Become a physiotherapist*. https://www.csp.org.uk/careers-jobs/what-physiotherapy.
78. Polston, G., R., S. Wallace, M., S., (2017). Chapter 67 - Analgesic Agents in Rheumatic Disease, *Kelley and Firestein's Textbook of Rheumatology (Tenth Edition),* 1075-1095, https://doi.org/10.1016/B978-0-323-31696-5.00067-X.

References – Chapter 7

1. Cerdá, B., Pérez, M., Pérez-Santiago, J. D., Tornero-Aguilera, J. F., González-Soltero, R., & Larrosa, M. (2016). Gut Microbiota Modification: Another Piece in the Puzzle of the Benefits of Physical Exercise in Health?. *Frontiers in physiology,* 7, 51. https://doi.org/10.3389/fphys.2016.00051

2. Codella, R., Luzi, L., & Terruzzi, I. (2018). Exercise has the guts: How physical activity may positively modulate gut microbiota in chronic and immune-based diseases. *Digestive and liver disease : official journal of the Italian Society of Gastroenterology and the Italian Association for the Study of the Liver*, *50*(4), 331–341. https://doi.org/10.1016/j.dld.2017.11.016.
3. University of California - San Diego. (2017, January 12). Exercise ... It does a body good: 20 minutes can act as anti-inflammatory: One moderate exercise session has a cellular response that may help suppress inflammation in the body. *ScienceDaily*. Retrieved August 20, 2020 from www.sciencedaily.com/releases/2017/01/170112115722.htm
4. Benatti, F. B., & Pedersen, B. K. (2015). Exercise as an anti-inflammatory therapy for rheumatic diseases-myokine regulation. *Nature reviews. Rheumatology*, *11*(2), 86–97. https://doi.org/10.1038/nrrheum.2014.193.
5. George, M. D., Giles, J. T., Katz, P. P., England, B. R., Mikuls, T. R., Michaud, K., Ogdie-Beatty, A. R., Ibrahim, S., Cannon, G. W., Caplan, L., Sauer, B. C., & Baker, J. F. (2017). Impact of Obesity and Adiposity on Inflammatory Markers in Patients With Rheumatoid Arthritis. Arthritis care & research, 69(12), 1789–1798. https://doi.org/10.1002/acr.23229.
6. Phillips, C. M., Dillon, C. B., & Perry, I. J. (2017). Does replacing sedentary behaviour with light or moderate to vigorous physical activity modulate inflammatory status in adults?. The international journal of behavioral nutrition and physical activity, 14(1), 138. https://doi.org/10.1186/s12966-017-0594-8.
7. Jankord, R., & Jemiolo, B. (2004). Influence of physical activity on serum IL-6 and IL-10 levels in healthy older men. *Medicine and science in sports and exercise*, *36*(6), 960–964. https://doi.org/10.1249/01.mss.0000128186.09416.18.
8. Iversen, M. D., Frits, M., von Heideken, J., Cui, J., Weinblatt, M., & Shadick, N. A. (2017). Physical Activity and Correlates of Physical Activity Participation Over Three Years in Adults With Rheumatoid Arthritis. *Arthritis care & research*, *69*(10), 1535–1545. https://doi.org/10.1002/acr.23156.
9. Summers, G., Booth, A., Brooke-Wavell, K., Barami, T., & Clemes, S. (2019). Physical activity and sedentary behavior in women with rheumatoid arthritis: a comparison of patients with low and high disease activity and healthy controls. *Open access rheumatology : research and reviews*, *11*, 133–142. https://doi.org/10.2147/OARRR.S203511.
10. Göksel Karatepe, A., Günaydin, R., Türkmen, G., & Kaya, T. (2011). Effects of home-based exercise program on the functional status and the quality of life in patients with rheumatoid arthritis: 1-year follow-up study. Rheumatology international, 31(2), 171–176. https://doi.org/10.1007/s00296-009-1242-7.

11. Veldhuijzen van Zanten, J. J., Rouse, P. C., Hale, E. D., Ntoumanis, N., Metsios, G. S., Duda, J. L., & Kitas, G. D. (2015). Perceived Barriers, Facilitators and Benefits for Regular Physical Activity and Exercise in Patients with Rheumatoid Arthritis: A Review of the Literature. *Sports medicine (Auckland, N.Z.)*, *45*(10), 1401–1412. https://doi.org/10.1007/s40279-015-0363-2.
12. Ytterberg, S., R., Mahowald, M., L., Krug, H.E. (1994). Exercise for arthritis, *Baillière's Clinical Rheumatology*, 8(1): 161-189, https://doi.org/10.1016/S0950-3579(05)80230-4.
13. Gleeson, M., Bishop, N. C., Stensel, D. J., Lindley, M. R., Mastana, S. S., & Nimmo, M. A. (2011). The anti-inflammatory effects of exercise: mechanisms and implications for the prevention and treatment of disease. Nature reviews. Immunology, 11(9), 607–615. https://doi.org/10.1038/nri3041.
14. Perandini, L. A., de Sá-Pinto, A. L., Roschel, H., Benatti, F. B., Lima, F. R., Bonfá, E., & Gualano, B. (2012). Exercise as a therapeutic tool to counteract inflammation and clinical symptoms in autoimmune rheumatic diseases. *Autoimmunity reviews*, *12*(2), 218–224. https://doi.org/10.1016/j.autrev.2012.06.007.
15. Lo, G, Driban, J, Kriska, A, Storti, K, McAlindon, T, Souza, T, Eaton, C, Petersen, N, Suarez-Almazor, M. (2014). Habitual running any time in life is not detrimental and may be protective of symptomatic knee osteoarthritis, *Arthritis and Rheumatology*, 2895.
16. Rausch Osthoff, A. K., Niedermann, K., Braun, J., Adams, J., Brodin, N., Dagfinrud, H., Duruoz, T., Esbensen, B. A., Günther, K. P., Hurkmans, E., Juhl, C. B., Kennedy, N., Kiltz, U., Knittle, K., Nurmohamed, M., Pais, S., Severijns, G., Swinnen, T. W., Pitsillidou, I. A., Warburton, L., … Vliet Vlieland, T. (2018). 2018 EULAR recommendations for physical activity in people with inflammatory arthritis and osteoarthritis. Annals of the rheumatic diseases, 77(9), 1251–1260. https://doi.org/10.1136/annrheumdis-2018-213585.
17. Kelley, G. A., Kelley, K. S., & Hootman, J. M. (2015). Effects of exercise on depression in adults with arthritis: a systematic review with meta-analysis of randomized controlled trials. Arthritis research & therapy, 17(1), 21. https://doi.org/10.1186/s13075-015-0533-5.
18. Warburton, D. E., Nicol, C. W., & Bredin, S. S. (2006). Health benefits of physical activity: the evidence. *CMAJ : Canadian Medical Association journal = journal de l'Association medicale canadienne*, *174*(6), 801–809. https://doi.org/10.1503/cmaj.051351.
19. Kramer A. (2020). An Overview of the Beneficial Effects of Exercise on Health and Performance. *Advances in experimental medicine and biology*, *1228*, 3–22. https://doi.org/10.1007/978-981-15-1792-1_1.

20. Reiner, M., Niermann, C., Jekauc, D., & Woll, A. (2013). Long-term health benefits of physical activity--a systematic review of longitudinal studies. BMC public health, 13, 813. https://doi.org/10.1186/1471-2458-13-813.
21. Løppenthin, K., Esbensen, B. A., Jennum, P., Østergaard, M., Christensen, J. F., Thomsen, T., Bech, J. S., & Midtgaard, J. (2014). Effect of intermittent aerobic exercise on sleep quality and sleep disturbances in patients with rheumatoid arthritis - design of a randomized controlled trial. BMC musculoskeletal disorders, 15, 49. https://doi.org/10.1186/1471-2474-15-49.
22. Zamani Sani, S. H., Fathirezaie, Z., Brand, S., Pühse, U., Holsboer-Trachsler, E., Gerber, M., & Talepasand, S. (2016). Physical activity and self-esteem: testing direct and indirect relationships associated with psychological and physical mechanisms. *Neuropsychiatric disease and treatment*, 12, 2617–2625. https://doi.org/10.2147/NDT.S116811.
23. Codella, R., Luzi, L., & Terruzzi, I. (2018). Exercise has the guts: How physical activity may positively modulate gut microbiota in chronic and immune-based diseases. *Digestive and liver disease: official journal of the Italian Society of Gastroenterology and the Italian Association for the Study of the Liver*, 50(4), 331–341. https://doi.org/10.1016/j.dld.2017.11.016.

References – Chapter 8

1. Colten, H. R., Altevogt, B. M., & Institute of Medicine (US) Committee on Sleep Medicine and Research (Eds.). (2006). Sleep Disorders and Sleep Deprivation: An Unmet Public Health Problem, 2 - Sleep Physiology. *National Academies Press (US)*. https://www.ncbi.nlm.nih.gov/books/NBK19956/.
2. Lyon L. (2019). Is an epidemic of sleeplessness increasing the incidence of Alzheimer's disease? *Brain : a journal of neurology*, 142(6), e30. https://doi.org/10.1093/brain/awz087.
3. Morin, C. M., LeBlanc, M., Daley, M., Gregoire, J. P., & Mérette, C. (2006). Epidemiology of insomnia: prevalence, self-help treatments, consultations, and determinants of help-seeking behaviors. Sleep medicine, 7(2), 123–130. https://doi.org/10.1016/j.sleep.2005.08.008.
4. Smith, M., T, Haythornthwaite, J., A. (2004). How do sleep disturbance and chronic pain inter-relate? Insights from the longitudinal and cognitive-behavioral clinical trials literature. *Sleep medicine reviews:* 8(2): 119-32. https://doi.org/10.1016/S1087-0792(03)00044-3.
5. Arthritis Foundation. Sleep and Pain. *Arthritis Foundation*. https://www.arthritis.org/health-wellness/healthy-living/managing-pain/fatigue-sleep/sleep-and-pain.

6. Walker, M. (2006). Sleep to Remember: The brain needs sleep before and after learning new things, regardless of the type of memory. Naps can help, but caffeine isn't an effective substitute. *American Scientist, 94*(4), 326-333. Retrieved July 19, 2020, from www.jstor.org/stable/27858801.
7. Finan, P. H., Goodin, B. R., & Smith, M. T. (2013). The association of sleep and pain: an update and a path forward. *The journal of pain : official journal of the American Pain Society,* 14(12), 1539–1552. https://doi.org/10.1016/j.jpain.2013.08.007.
8. Koffel, E., Kroenke, K., Bair, M. J., Leverty, D., Polusny, M. A., & Krebs, E. E. (2016). The bidirectional relationship between sleep complaints and pain: Analysis of data from a randomized trial. *Health Psychology,* 35(1), 41–49. https://doi.org/10.1037/hea0000245.
9. Haack, M., Simpson, N., Sethna, N., Kaur, S., & Mullington, J. (2020). Sleep deficiency and chronic pain: potential underlying mechanisms and clinical implications. *Neuropsychopharmacology : official publication of the American College of Neuropsychopharmacology,* 45(1), 205–216. https://doi.org/10.1038/s41386-019-0439-z.
10. Irwin, M. R., Olmstead, R., Carrillo, C., Sadeghi, N., Fitzgerald, J. D., Ranganath, V. K., & Nicassio, P. M. (2012). Sleep loss exacerbates fatigue, depression, and pain in rheumatoid arthritis. *Sleep,* 35(4), 537–543. https://doi.org/10.5665/sleep.1742.
11. Smith, M. T., Edwards, R. R., McCann, U. D., & Haythornthwaite, J. A. (2007). The effects of sleep deprivation on pain inhibition and spontaneous pain in women. *Sleep,* 30(4), 494–505. https://doi.org/10.1093/sleep/30.4.494.
12. Roehrs, T., & Roth, T. (2005). Sleep and pain: interaction of two vital functions. Seminars in neurology, 25(1), 106–116. https://doi.org/10.1055/s-2005-867079.
13. Walker, M. (2018). *Why We Sleep: The New Science of Sleep and Dreams.* London: Penguin Random House.
14. Bryant, P. A., Trinder, J., & Curtis, N. (2004). Sick and tired: Does sleep have a vital role in the immune system?. Nature reviews. *Immunology,* 4(6), 457–467. https://doi.org/10.1038/nri1369.
15. Prather, A. A., Janicki-Deverts, D., Hall, M. H., & Cohen, S. (2015). Behaviorally Assessed Sleep and Susceptibility to the Common Cold. *Sleep,* 38(9), 1353–1359. https://doi.org/10.5665/sleep.4968.
16. Finan, P. H., Goodin, B. R., & Smith, M. T. (2013). The association of sleep and pain: an update and a path forward. *The journal of pain : official journal of the American Pain Society,* 14(12), 1539–1552. https://doi.org/10.1016/j.jpain.2013.08.007.

17. Hong, H., Maury, E. Ramsey, K., M., Perelis, M., Marcheva, B., Omura, C., Kobayashi, Y., Guttridge, D., C., Barish, G., D., Bass, J.. (2018). Requirement for NF-κB in maintenance of molecular and behavioral circadian rhythms in mice. *Genes & Development*, doi: 10.1101/gad.319228.118.
18. Solarz, D. E., Mullington, J. M., & Meier-Ewert, H. K. (2012). Sleep, inflammation and cardiovascular disease. Frontiers in bioscience (Elite edition), 4, 2490–2501. https://doi.org/10.2741/e560.
19. Irwin, M. R., Wang, M., Campomayor, C. O., Collado-Hidalgo, A., & Cole, S. (2006). Sleep deprivation and activation of morning levels of cellular and genomic markers of inflammation. Archives of internal medicine, 166(16), 1756–1762. https://doi.org/10.1001/archinte.166.16.1756.
20. Irwin, M. R., Wang, M., Ribeiro, D., Cho, H. J., Olmstead, R., Breen, E. C., Martinez-Maza, O., & Cole, S. (2008). Sleep loss activates cellular inflammatory signaling. Biological psychiatry, 64(6), 538–540. https://doi.org/10.1016/j.biopsych.2008.05.004.
21. Youm, Y. H., Nguyen, K. Y., Grant, R. W., Goldberg, E. L., Bodogai, M., Kim, D., D'Agostino, D., Planavsky, N., Lupfer, C., Kanneganti, T. D., Kang, S., Horvath, T. L., Fahmy, T. M., Crawford, P. A., Biragyn, A., Alnemri, E., & Dixit, V. D. (2015). The ketone metabolite β-hydroxybutyrate blocks NLRP3 inflammasome-mediated inflammatory disease. Nature medicine, 21(3), 263–269. https://doi.org/10.1038/nm.3804.
22. Hauri P. (1977). Sleep hygiene. *Current Concepts: The Sleep Disorders*. The Upjohn Company; Kalamazoo, MI: 21–35.
23. Zarcone VP. (2000). Sleep hygiene. *Principles and Practice of Sleep Medicine*. 3rd ed. WB Saunders; Philadelphia, PA: 657–61.
24. Yahia, N., Brown, C., Potter, S., Szymanski, H., Smith, K., Pringle, L., Herman, C., Uribe, M., Fu, Z., Chung, M., & Geliebter, A. (2017). Night eating syndrome and its association with weight status, physical activity, eating habits, smoking status, and sleep patterns among college students. *Eating and weight disorders : EWD*, *22*(3), 421–433. https://doi.org/10.1007/s40519-017-0403-z.
25. O'Reardon, J. P., Ringel, B. L., Dinges, D. F., Allison, K. C., Rogers, N. L., Martino, N. S., & Stunkard, A. J. (2004). Circadian eating and sleeping patterns in the night eating syndrome. *Obesity research*, *12*(11), 1789–1796. https://doi.org/10.1038/oby.2004.222.
26. Fujiwara, Y., Machida, A., Watanabe, Y., Shiba, M., Tominaga, K., Watanabe, T., Oshitani, N., Higuchi, K., & Arakawa, T. (2005). Association between dinner-to-bed time and gastro-esophageal reflux disease. *The American journal of gastroenterology*, *100*(12), 2633–2636. https://doi.org/10.1111/j.1572-0241.2005.00354.x.

27. Gill, S., & Panda, S. (2015). A Smartphone App Reveals Erratic Diurnal Eating Patterns in Humans that Can Be Modulated for Health Benefits. Cell metabolism, 22(5), 789–798. https://doi.org/10.1016/j.cmet.2015.09.005.
28. Roehrs, Timothy, and Thomas Roth. (2008). Caffeine: sleep and daytime sleepiness. *Sleep medicine reviews*. 12(2): 153-62. https://doi.org/10.1016/j.smrv.2007.07.004.
29. M. H. Bonnet, D. L. Arand (1992). Caffeine Use as a Model of Acute and Chronic Insomnia, *Sleep*, 15(6): 526–536, https://doi.org/10.1093/sleep/15.6.526.
30. Dunwiddie, T. V., & Masino, S. A. (2001). The role and regulation of adenosine in the central nervous system. Annual review of neuroscience, 24, 31–55. https://doi.org/10.1146/annurev.neuro.24.1.31.
31. Ferré S. (2008). An update on the mechanisms of the psychostimulant effects of caffeine. Journal of neurochemistry, 105(4), 1067–1079. https://doi.org/10.1111/j.1471-4159.2007.05196.x.
32. Drake, C., Roehrs, T., Shambroom, J., & Roth, T. (2013). Caffeine effects on sleep taken 0, 3, or 6 hours before going to bed. Journal of clinical sleep medicine : JCSM : official publication of the American Academy of Sleep Medicine, 9(11), 1195–1200. https://doi.org/10.5664/jcsm.3170.
33. Ganesh, J. (2019, January 11). Sleep expert Matthew Walker on the secret to a good night's rest. *Financial Times*. https://www.ft.com/content/e6ccdcac-133d-11e9-a581-4ff78404524e.
34. Colrain, I. M., Nicholas, C. L., & Baker, F. C. (2014). Alcohol and the sleeping brain. *Handbook of clinical neurology*, *125*, 415–431. https://doi.org/10.1016/B978-0-444-62619-6.00024-0.
35. Loprinzi, P., D., Cardinal, B., J. (2011). Association between objectively-measured physical activity and sleep, NHANES 2005–2006. *Mental Health and Physical Activity*, 4 (2): 65 doi: 10.1016/j.mhpa.2011.08.001.
36. Blume, C., Garbazza, C., & Spitschan, M. (2019). Effects of light on human circadian rhythms, sleep and mood. *Somnologie : Schlafforschung und Schlafmedizin = Somnology : sleep research and sleep medicine*, *23*(3), 147–156. https://doi.org/10.1007/s11818-019-00215-x.
37. Gao, Q., Kou, T., Zhuang, B., Ren, Y., Dong, X., & Wang, Q. (2018). The Association between Vitamin D Deficiency and Sleep Disorders: A Systematic Review and Meta-Analysis. *Nutrients*, *10*(10), 1395. https://doi.org/10.3390/nu10101395.
38. McCarty, D., E., Chesson, A., L., Jain, S., K., Marino, A., A. (2014). The link between vitamin D metabolism and sleep medicine, *Sleep Medicine Reviews*, 18(4): 311-319, https://doi.org/10.1016/j.smrv.2013.07.001.
39. Yetish, G., Kaplan, H., Gurven, M., Wood, B., Pontzer, H., Manger, P. R., Wilson, C., McGregor, R., & Siegel, J. M. (2015). Natural sleep and

its seasonal variations in three pre-industrial societies. *Current biology : CB*, *25*(21), 2862–2868. https://doi.org/10.1016/j.cub.2015.09.046.

40. Chang, A. M., Aeschbach, D., Duffy, J. F., & Czeisler, C. A. (2015). Evening use of light-emitting eReaders negatively affects sleep, circadian timing, and next-morning alertness. *Proceedings of the National Academy of Sciences of the United States of America*, 112(4), 1232–1237. https://doi.org/10.1073/pnas.1418490112.
41. Afolalu, E. F., Moore, C., Ramlee, F., Goodchild, C. E., & Tang, N. K. (2016). Development of the Pain-Related Beliefs and Attitudes about Sleep (PBAS) Scale for the Assessment and Treatment of Insomnia Comorbid with Chronic Pain. *Journal of clinical sleep medicine : JCSM: official publication of the American Academy of Sleep Medicine*, *12*(9), 1269–1277. https://doi.org/10.5664/jcsm.6130.
42. Ackerley R, Badre G, Olausson H (2015) Positive Effects of a Weighted Blanket on Insomnia. *J Sleep Med Disord* 2(3): 1022. Accessed via: https://www.jscimedcentral.com/SleepMedicine/sleepmedicine-2-1022.pdf.
43. Murphy, P. J., & Campbell, S. S. (1997). Nighttime drop in body temperature: a physiological trigger for sleep onset?. *Sleep*, *20*(7), 505–511. https://doi.org/10.1093/sleep/20.7.505.
44. Meng, X., Li, Y., Li, S., Zhou, Y., Gan, R. Y., Xu, D. P., & Li, H. B. (2017). Dietary Sources and Bioactivities of Melatonin. *Nutrients*, *9*(4), 367. https://doi.org/10.3390/nu9040367.
45. Kapalka, G., M. (2010). Chapter 4 - Substances Involved in Neurotransmission, Practical Resources for the Mental Health Professional, *Nutritional and Herbal Therapies for Children and Adolescents*, 71-99, https://doi.org/10.1016/B978-0-12-374927-7.00004-2.
46. Srivastava, J. K., Shankar, E., & Gupta, S. (2010). Chamomile: A herbal medicine of the past with bright future. *Molecular medicine reports*, *3*(6), 895–901. https://doi.org/10.3892/mmr.2010.377.
47. Chang, S. M., & Chen, C. H. (2016). Effects of an intervention with drinking chamomile tea on sleep quality and depression in sleep disturbed postnatal women: a randomized controlled trial. *Journal of advanced nursing*, 72(2), 306–315. https://doi.org/10.1111/jan.12836.
48. Zick, S. M., Wright, B. D., Sen, A., & Arnedt, J. T. (2011). Preliminary examination of the efficacy and safety of a standardized chamomile extract for chronic primary insomnia: a randomized placebo-controlled pilot study. *BMC complementary and alternative medicine*, *11*, 78. https://doi.org/10.1186/1472-6882-11-78.
49. Fernández-San-Martín, M. I., Masa-Font, R., Palacios-Soler, L., Sancho-Gómez, P., Calbó-Caldentey, C., & Flores-Mateo, G.

(2010). Effectiveness of Valerian on insomnia: a meta-analysis of randomized placebo-controlled trials. *Sleep medicine*, *11*(6), 505–511. https://doi.org/10.1016/j.sleep.2009.12.009.

50. Ngan, A., & Conduit, R. (2011). A double-blind, placebo-controlled investigation of the effects of *Passiflora incarnata* (passionflower) herbal tea on subjective sleep quality. *Phytotherapy research : PTR*, *25*(8), 1153–1159. https://doi.org/10.1002/ptr.3400.
51. Elsas, S. M., Rossi, D. J., Raber, J., White, G., Seeley, C. A., Gregory, W. L., Mohr, C., Pfankuch, T., & Soumyanath, A. (2010). *Passiflora incarnata* L. (Passionflower) extracts elicit GABA currents in hippocampal neurons in vitro, and show anxiogenic and anticonvulsant effects in vivo, varying with extraction method. *Phytomedicine : international journal of phytotherapy and phytopharmacology*, *17*(12), 940–949. https://doi.org/10.1016/j.phymed.2010.03.002.
52. Cases, J., Ibarra, A., Feuillère, N., Roller, M., & Sukkar, S. G. (2011). Pilot trial of *Melissa officinalis* L. leaf extract in the treatment of volunteers suffering from mild-to-moderate anxiety disorders and sleep disturbances. *Mediterranean journal of nutrition and metabolism*, *4*(3), 211–218. https://doi.org/10.1007/s12349-010-0045-4.
53. Yoo, D. Y., Choi, J. H., Kim, W., Yoo, K. Y., Lee, C. H., Yoon, Y. S., Won, M. H., & Hwang, I. K. (2011). Effects of *Melissa officinalis* L. (lemon balm) extract on neurogenesis associated with serum corticosterone and GABA in the mouse dentate gyrus. Neurochemical research, 36(2), 250–257. https://doi.org/10.1007/s11064-010-0312-2.
54. Chumpitazi, B. P., Kearns, G. L., & Shulman, R. J. (2018). Review article: the physiological effects and safety of peppermint oil and its efficacy in irritable bowel syndrome and other functional disorders. *Alimentary pharmacology & therapeutics*, *47*(6), 738–752. https://doi.org/10.1111/apt.14519.
55. Koulivand, P. H., Khaleghi Ghadiri, M., & Gorji, A. (2013). Lavender and the nervous system. *Evidence-based complementary and alternative medicine : eCAM*, *2013*, 681304. https://doi.org/10.1155/2013/681304.
56. Keshavarz Afshar, M., Behboodi Moghadam, Z., Taghizadeh, Z., Bekhradi, R., Montazeri, A., & Mokhtari, P. (2015). Lavender fragrance essential oil and the quality of sleep in postpartum women. *Iranian Red Crescent medical journal*, *17*(4), e25880. https://doi.org/10.5812/ircmj.17(4)2015.25880.
57. Lillehei, A. S., Halcón, L. L., Savik, K., & Reis, R. (2015). Effect of Inhaled Lavender and Sleep Hygiene on Self-Reported Sleep Issues: A Randomized Controlled Trial. *Journal of alternative and complementary medicine (New York, N.Y.)*, *21*(7), 430–438. https://doi.org/10.1089/acm.2014.0327.

58. Karadag, E., Samancioglu, S., Ozden, D., & Bakir, E. (2017). Effects of aromatherapy on sleep quality and anxiety of patients. *Nursing in critical care*, *22*(2), 105–112. https://doi.org/10.1111/nicc.12198.
59. Chen, S. L., & Chen, C. H. (2015). Effects of Lavender Tea on Fatigue, Depression, and Maternal-Infant Attachment in Sleep-Disturbed Postnatal Women. *Worldviews on evidence-based nursing*, *12*(6), 370–379. https://doi.org/10.1111/wvn.12122.

References – Chapter 9

1. Briggs, A. M., Cross, M. J., Hoy, D. G., Sànchez-Riera, L., Blyth, F. M., Woolf, A. D., & March, L. (2016). Musculoskeletal Health Conditions Represent a Global Threat to Healthy Aging: A Report for the 2015 World Health Organization World Report on Ageing and Health. The Gerontologist, 56 Suppl 2, S243–S255. https://doi.org/10.1093/geront/gnw002.
2. Lépine, J. P., & Briley, M. (2004). The epidemiology of pain in depression. Human psychopharmacology, 19 Suppl 1, S3–S7. https://doi.org/10.1002/hup.618.
3. Public Health England. (2018). PHE Fingertips Tool Musculoskeletal Disease Profile. *Public Health England*.
4. García H., and Miralles F. (2016). *Ikigai: The Japanese Secret to a Long and Happy Life*. London: Hutchinson.
5. Liu, Y. Z., Wang, Y. X., & Jiang, C. L. (2017). Inflammation: The Common Pathway of Stress-Related Diseases. *Frontiers in human neuroscience*, *11*, 316. https://doi.org/10.3389/fnhum.2017.00316.
1. Pittenger, C., Duman, R. (2008). Stress, Depression, and Neuroplasticity: A Convergence of Mechanisms. *Neuropsychopharmacol* 33, 88–109. https://doi.org/10.1038/sj.npp.1301574.
1. Danese, A., Moffitt, T. E., Harrington, H., Milne, B. J., Polanczyk, G., Pariante, C. M., Poulton, R., & Caspi, A. (2009). Adverse childhood experiences and adult risk factors for age-related disease: depression, inflammation, and clustering of metabolic risk markers. Archives of pediatrics & adolescent medicine, 163(12), 1135–1143. https://doi.org/10.1001/archpediatrics.2009.214.
1. Carnegie Mellon University. (2012, April 2). How stress influences disease: Study reveals inflammation as the culprit. ScienceDaily. Retrieved November 23, 2020 from www.sciencedaily.com/releases/2012/04/120402162546.htm.
1. Harrison, N. A., Brydon, L., Walker, C., Gray, M. A., Steptoe, A., & Critchley, H. D. (2009). Inflammation causes mood changes through alterations

in subgenual cingulate activity and mesolimbic connectivity. *Biological psychiatry*, 66(5), 407–414. https://doi.org/10.1016/j.biopsych.2009.03.015.

2. Edward Bullmore. E., (2018). *The Inflamed Mind: A Radical New Approach to Depression*. London: Short Books.
3. Kohler, O., Krogh, J., Mors, O., & Benros, M. E. (2016). Inflammation in Depression and the Potential for Anti-Inflammatory Treatment. *Current neuropharmacology*, *14*(7), 732–742. https://doi.org/10.2174/1570159x14666151208113700.
4. Devore, Elizabeth & Kang, Jae & Breteler, Monique & Grodstein, Francine. (2012). Dietary Intakes of Berries and Flavonoids in Relation to Cognitive Decline. *Annals of neurology.* 72. 135-43. 10.1002/ana.23594.
5. Ng, T. P., Chiam, P. C., Lee, T., Chua, H. C., Lim, L., & Kua, E. H. (2006). Curry consumption and cognitive function in the elderly. *American journal of epidemiology*, *164*(9), 898–906. https://doi.org/10.1093/aje/kwj267.
6. Foster H (2019, October), The diet to tame inflammation. *Women's Health Magazine,* pp.48-50.
7. Jacka, F. N., Ystrom, E., Brantsaeter, A. L., Karevold, E., Roth, C., Haugen, M., Meltzer, H. M., Schjolberg, S., & Berk, M. (2013). Maternal and early postnatal nutrition and mental health of offspring by age 5 years: a prospective cohort study. Journal of the American Academy of Child and Adolescent Psychiatry, 52(10), 1038–1047. https://doi.org/10.1016/j.jaac.2013.07.002.
8. Jacka, F. N., Mykletun, A., Berk, M., Bjelland, I., & Tell, G. S. (2011). The association between habitual diet quality and the common mental disorders in community-dwelling adults: the Hordaland Health study. *Psychosomatic medicine*, *73*(6), 483–490. https://doi.org/10.1097/PSY.0b013e318222831a.
9. Pennisi, E. (2020, May 7). Meet the 'psychobiome': the gut bacteria that may alter how you think, feel, and act. *Science*. doi:10.1126/science.abc6637.
10. Versus Arthritis. (2018, November). Defying Arthritis at Every Age Report. *Versus Arthritis*. https://www.versusarthritis.org/media/2461/defying_arthritis_at_every_age-report-nov-18.pdf.
11. Bower, J. E., Irwin, M., R. (2016). Mind–body therapies and control of inflammatory biology: A descriptive review, *Brain, Behavior, and Immunity*, 51: 1-11, https://doi.org/10.1016/j.bbi.2015.06.012.
12. Saeed, S. A., Cunningham, K., & Bloch, R. M. (2019). Depression and Anxiety Disorders: Benefits of Exercise, Yoga, and Meditation. *American family physician*, *99*(10), 620–627.
13. McMahan, D., L., Braun, E. (2017). *Meditation, Buddhism, and Science*. New York: Oxford University Press.
14. Goodreads. Alice Morse Earle Quotes. *Goodreads.com*. https://www.goodreads.com/author/quotes/44874.Alice_Morse_Earle.

15. Zak, P. (2014, April 22). Dogs (and Cats) Can Love. *The Atlantic*. https://www.theatlantic.com/health/archive/2014/04/does-your-dog-or-cat-actually-love-you/360784/.
16. Beetz, A., Uvnäs-Moberg, K., Julius, H., & Kotrschal, K. (2012). Psychosocial and psychophysiological effects of human-animal interactions: the possible role of oxytocin. *Frontiers in psychology*, *3*, 234. https://doi.org/10.3389/fpsyg.2012.00234.
17. Gullone, E. (2000). The Biophilia Hypothesis and Life in the 21st Century: Increasing Mental Health or Increasing Pathology?. *Journal of Happiness Studies*, 1, 293–322. https://doi.org/10.1023/A:1010043827986.
18. Farrow, M. R., & Washburn, K. (2019). A Review of Field Experiments on the Effect of Forest Bathing on Anxiety and Heart Rate Variability. *Global advances in health and medicine*, *8*, 2164956119848654. https://doi.org/10.1177/2164956119848654.
19. Hansen, M. M., Jones, R., & Tocchini, K. (2017). Shinrin-Yoku (Forest Bathing) and Nature Therapy: A State-of-the-Art Review. *International journal of environmental research and public health*, *14*(8), 851. https://doi.org/10.3390/ijerph14080851.
20. Igarashi, M., Song, C., Ikei, H., & Miyazaki, Y. (2015). Effect of stimulation by foliage plant display images on prefrontal cortex activity: a comparison with stimulation using actual foliage plants. *Journal of neuroimaging : official journal of the American Society of Neuroimaging*, *25*(1), 127–130. https://doi.org/10.1111/jon.12078.
21. Lewis, D. (2009). 'Galaxy Stress Research'. *Mindlab International, Sussex University*. Accessed: http://nationalreadingcampaign.ca/wp-content/uploads/2013/09/ReadingFacts1.pdf.
22. Smith, M. A., Thompson, A., Hall, L. J., Allen, S. F., & Wetherell, M. A. (2018). The physical and psychological health benefits of positive emotional writing: Investigating the moderating role of Type D (distressed) personality. *British journal of health psychology*, *23*(4), 857–871. https://doi.org/10.1111/bjhp.12320.
23. Kaimal, G., Ray, K., & Muniz, J. (2016). Reduction of Cortisol Levels and Participants' Responses Following Art Making. *Art therapy: journal of the American Art Therapy Association*, *33*(2), 74–80. https://doi.org/10.1080/07421656.2016.1166832.
24. Kaimal, G., Ayaz, H., Herres, J., Dieterich-Hartwell, R., Makwana, B., Kaiser, D., H., Nasser, J., A. (2017). Functional near-infrared spectroscopy assessment of reward perception based on visual self-expression: Coloring, doodling, and free drawing. *The Arts in Psychotherapy*, *55*(85). doi: 10.1016/j.aip.2017.05.004.

25. Reynolds, F., & Prior, S. (2003). 'A lifestyle coat-hanger': a phenomenological study of the meanings of artwork for women coping with chronic illness and disability. *Disability and rehabilitation*, *25*(14), 785–794. https://doi.org/10.1080/0963828031000093486.
26. Mendick, R. (2011, May 8). *Brain Scans Reveal the Power of Art*. The Telegraph. https://www.telegraph.co.uk/culture/art/art-news/8500012/Brain-scans-reveal-the-power-of-art.html.
27. Melua, K. (2005). Spider's Web [Recorded by Katie Melua.]. On *Piece by Piece*. [MP3 file]. London, England: Dramatico Records.
28. Leubner, D., & Hinterberger, T. (2017). Reviewing the Effectiveness of Music Interventions in Treating Depression. *Frontiers in psychology*, *8*, 1109. https://doi.org/10.3389/fpsyg.2017.01109.
29. Ekholm, O., Juel, K., & Bonde, L. O. (2016). Associations between daily musicking and health: Results from a nationwide survey in Denmark. *Scandinavian journal of public health*, *44*(7), 726–732. https://doi.org/10.1177/1403494816664252.
30. Pascoe, M. C., Thompson, D. R., & Ski, C. F. (2017). Yoga, mindfulness-based stress reduction and stress-related physiological measures: A meta-analysis. *Psychoneuroendocrinology*, *86*, 152–168. https://doi.org/10.1016/j.psyneuen.2017.08.008.
31. Urban Dictionary. (2018, November 17). *Definition: "I'm fine."*. https://www.urbandictionary.com/define.php?term=I%27m%20fine.
32. Oprah Winfrey [@Oprah]. (2015, April, 12). "As long as you are breathing there is more right with you than wrong with you , no matter what is wrong" #SuperSoulSunday [Tweet]. Twitter. https://twitter.com/Oprah/status/587277611723665408?s=20.

Conversion Chart

Metric/Imperial/US Conversion Chart

All equivalents are rounded, for practical convenience.

Weight

25g	1 oz
50g	2 oz
100g	3½ oz
150g	5 oz
200g	7 oz
250g	9 oz
300g	10 oz
400g	14 oz
500g	1 lb 2 oz
1 kg	2¼ lb

Volume (liquids)

5ml		1 tsp
15ml		1 tbsp
30ml	1 fl oz	2 tbsp
60ml	2 fl oz	¼ cup
75ml		⅓ cup
120ml	4 fl oz	½ cup
150ml	5 fl oz	⅔ cup
175ml		¾ cup
250ml	8 fl oz	1 cup
1 litre	1 quart	4 cups

Volume (dry ingredients – an approximate guide)

butter	1 cup (2 sticks) = 225g
rolled oats	1 cup = 100g
fine powders (e.g. flour)	1 cup = 125g
breadcrumbs (fresh)	1 cup = 50g
breadcrumbs (dried)	1 cup = 125g
nuts (e.g. almonds)	1 cup = 125g
seeds (e.g. chia)	1 cup = 160g
dried fruit (e.g. raisins)	1 cup = 150g
dried legumes (large, e.g. chickpeas)	1 cup = 170g
grains, granular goods and small dried legumes (e.g. rice, quinoa, sugar, lentils)	1 cup = 200g
grated cheese	1 cup = 100g

Length

1cm	½ inch
2.5cm	1 inch
20cm	8 inches
25cm	10 inches
30cm	12 inches

Oven temperatures

Celsius	**Fahrenheit**
140	275
150	300
160	325
180	350
190	375
200	400
220	425
230	450

Index

About the Author

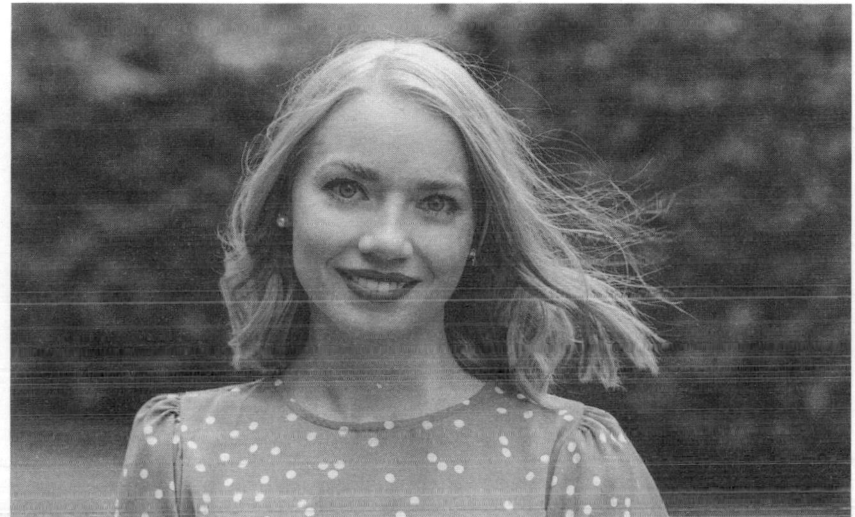

Photograph by Louise Rose Photography

Emily Johnson launched the Instagram page @arthritisfoodie in September 2018 after struggling with seronegative arthritis for five years. The page has since gained more than 10k followers, with people looking to Emily for inspiration on living healthily with arthritis. Emily also works in marketing and is a social media influencer.

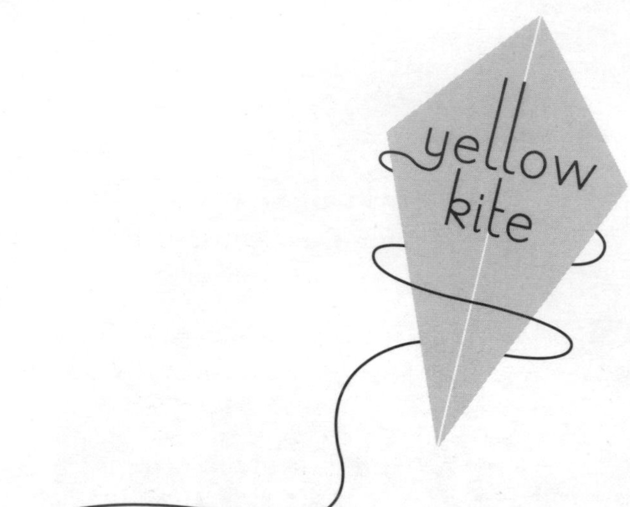

books to help you live a good life

Join the conversation and tell
us how you live a #goodlife

@yellowkitebooks

YellowKiteBooks

Yellow Kite Books

YellowKiteBooks